Edited by
J. K. WING

Health Services Planning and Research

Contributions from Psychiatric Case Registers

GASKELL

Typeset by Dobbie Typesetting Limited, Plymouth, Devon
Printed in Great Britain by Henry Ling Ltd, at the Dorset Press,
Dorchester, Dorset

Contents

List of registers   vii

Preface   ix

Part I. Introduction

1   Introduction to the registers and plan of the book   *J. K. Wing*   3

Part II. Statistics

2   In-patient statistics from eight psychiatric case registers, 1977–83 *C. Jennings, G. Der, C. Robinson, S. Rose, J. de Alarcon, D. Hunter, R. Holliday and N. Moss*   13

3   A decade of mental health care in an English urban community: patterns and trends in Salford, 1976–87   *T. Fryers and K. Wooff*   31

4   The effects of population changes on long-stay in-patient rates   *G. Der*   53

5   Powick Hospital, 1978–86: a case register study   *C. Hassall and S. Rose*   58

Part III. Comparative studies

6   Community psychiatric nursing services in Salford, Southampton and Worcester   *K. Wooff, S. Rose and J. Street*   73

7   The use of psychiatric services by the elderly: a study based on the case registers of Nottingham, Salford, Southampton and Worcester *S. Jones, C. Hassall, C. Jennings and M. Cleverly*   81

8   A five-year follow-up of deliberate self-poisoning in Oxford and Worcester   *J. de Alarcon, J. Fooks, C. Hassall and S. Rose*   94

Part IV. Future developments

9   The development of other European case registers   *G. H. M. M. ten Horn*   107

10 Some national and regional statistical challenges   *P. M. Williamson*   110
11 Information for planning: case registers and Körner   *J. E. Cooper*   115
12 The future of psychiatric case registers   *J. K. Wing*   121

List of registers

The people listed below were members of the Technical Committee and (in parentheses) of the Directors' Committee, which together comprised the joint UK Inter-register Committee.

Aberdeen: Mr D. Hunter, Department of Mental Health Research Unit, Aberdeen AB9 2ZX, tel. 0224 632391 (Dr C. McCance)

Camberwell: Mr G. Der, MRC Social Psychiatry Unit, London SE5 8AF, tel. 01 703 5411, ext. 3512 (Prof. J. K. Wing)

Cardiff: Mr N. Moss, Information Co-ordinating Centre for Mental Health, Whitchurch Hospital, Cardiff CF4 7XB, tel. 0222 693191, ext. 6366 (Dr A. Thomas, Chairman of Steering Committee)

Edinburgh: Ms S. Millar and Mrs R. Holliday, Andrew Duncan Clinic, Royal Edinburgh Hospital, Morningside Terrace, Edinburgh EH10 5HF, tel. 031 447 2011, ext. 4498 (Dr J. B. Loudon)

Nottingham: Mrs S. Jones (now Lecturer, Department of General Practice) and Mrs N. Davis, Professorial Unit, Mapperley Hospital, Nottingham NG3 6AA, tel. 0602 700111, ext. 417 (Prof. J. E. Cooper)

Oxford: Dr J. de Alarcon and Ms J. Fooks, Oxford Record Linkage Study, Oxford Regional Health Authority, Old Road, Headington, Oxford OX3 7LF, tel. 0865 64861, ext. 241

Salford: Dr K. Wooff, Ms C. Robinson and Mr M. Cleverly, Pendleton House, Broughton Road, Salford M6 6LQ, tel. 061 736 2673 and 2675 (Dr T. Fryers)

Southampton: Mr C. Jennings and Miss J. Street, for whom correspondence should be addressed to: University Department of Psychiatry, Southampton SO9 4PE (Prof. J. Gibbons)

Worcester: Dr C. Hassall and Mrs S. Rose, Department of Psychiatry, Queen Elizabeth Hospital, Birmingham B15 2TH, tel. 021 414 6874 (Prof. I. Brockington)

Other authors: Mrs P. M. Williamson, formerly of the Department of Health and Social Security
Dr G. H. M. M. ten Horn, Superintendent, Eemeroord, Zandheuvelweg 4, 3744, MM Baarn, The Netherlands; formerly of the Groningen Register, The Netherlands.

Preface

From 1980 to 1986 there were regular meetings of the joint UK Inter-register Committee (Chairman, Professor James Gibbons; Co-ordinator, Mr Christopher Jennings), which comprised the directors and the technical heads of nine psychiatric case registers covering areas in Great Britain. Details of membership are on the previous page. At the last of these meetings, members agreed to produce a monograph of statistics comparing the register areas with each other and with data for England, Scotland and Wales. Chapters describing research carried out on the basis of in the context of registers would also be provided. The work was finished and printed by the Department of Health and Social Security (DHSS) in 1987. However, because the edition was limited in number, and unlikely to be noticed because not formally published, it was decided that a publisher should be sought. The authors are very pleased that Gaskell agreed to accept it, and are grateful to the DHSS for a contribution to the costs.

Owing to pressures on its research budget, the DHSS withdrew its central funding from the Nottingham, Salford and Southampton registers, to which it had been giving substantial support, at the end of March 1987. This led to the closure of the Southampton register. The Nottingham and Salford registers were able to continue, funded by their health districts. The Worcester district health authority ceased funding its register in 1986. The Camberwell register, supported by the Medical Research Council, had closed in 1985. The other four registers continue to be funded by their local districts, with contributions from the regional health authority (Oxford), a local university and the Scottish Home and Health Department (Aberdeen).

National in-patient figures were obtained from the following sources:

England: *In-patient Statistics from the Mental Health Enquiry for England* (various years, HMSO), and *Statistical Notes, Statistical Bulletins* and personal communications from DHSS Statistics and Research Division 2C
Wales: personal communication, Welsh Office
Scotland: personal communication, Information Services Division, Common Services Agency, Edinburgh.

Our thanks are due to the clerical and computing staff of the registers, who collect and process the data, and to the health service and local authority staff on whose co-operation registers depend.

J. K. Wing

I. Introduction

1 Introduction to the registers and plan of the book

J. K. WING

Advantages and limitations

Psychiatric case registers are local information systems that record the contacts with designated social and medical services of patients or clients from a defined geographical area. This information is stored in a linked and cumulative file so that the care of any individual or group can be followed over time, no matter how complex the pattern of service attendance. Statistics can therefore be based on either people or events. The fact that registers are local and have specialist staff means that the information collected is of high quality. The geographical base allows rates to be calculated and epidemiological research to be conducted. If necessary, data can be collected concerning all users of any particular agency or service, including those who do not come from the local area. These characteristics ensure an excellent information base that can be used for several purposes. For most registers, a central purpose is to assist local planning.

In addition to these local functions, rates can be compared on the basis of service contacts and population characteristics. Statistics from a number of areas can complement the knowledge of psychiatric services available from national statistics or ad hoc studies. Register statistics are more detailed, comprehensive and reliable than national or district figures, and an examination of the similarities and differences between areas with known characteristics can put the results from one area into a wider perspective, help evaluate the local service, and improve understanding of how various patterns of services work.

Registers have a number of limitations. They collect information from specialist services and so do not include people treated only by general practitioners or those who receive no medical help at all. Migration into and out of the relatively small areas covered by most registers may be considerable. Because it is not known, without special follow-up, whether someone who ceases contact with a service agency has left the area or stopped attending for other reasons, the interpretation of results may be restricted. Nevertheless, within specified limits, registers do provide an important contribution to knowledge.

Inter-register collaboration

Producing comparable statistics from a number of registers presents problems because each has been developed to serve local as well as general purposes.

The services recorded are not identical in each area and data cannot be recorded in exactly the same way. The resources available to registers are not uniform. In spite of these difficulties, there have been substantial efforts to adopt similar definitions and practices. Several studies that present comparative statistics have been published (Bahn *et al*, 1966; Wing *et al*, 1967, 1972; Wing & Fryers, 1976). From quite early in the history of the UK registers it was customary to hold occasional inter-register meetings at which problems of comparability were discussed and data from various registers compared (Wing & Bransby, 1970; Department of Health and Social Security, 1974).

It was not, however, until 1980 that the eight UK registers then established began to hold regular meetings at least once or twice a year. These resulted in a set of statistics, with a brief commentary, that was published in mimeographed form (Gibbons *et al*, 1984). Like the earlier publication by Wing & Fryers (1976), there was a long-lasting, and to the authors surprising, demand that eventually almost exhausted the rather exiguous initial supply. It was decided, therefore, to provide a more readily available volume, based in part on an expansion of the earlier work, but adding chapters by groups of register workers who researched topics that their particular registers made especially suitable for investigation. Data from a ninth register, covering Edinburgh, have also been included.

Part of the material in the present chapter is edited from Chapters 1 and 2 of Gibbons *et al* (1984). Chapter 3 of that compilation contains material, particularly tables relating to day care, that is not used in this volume, but copies are still available.

Characteristics of the register areas

The areas in which the nine registers described in this report are situated are predominantly urban and therefore represent, between them, most, but not all, parts of the country. (The name used throughout the book for each register area is a conventional shorthand term–a formal description of the geographical areas is given by Gibbons *et al* (1984).) They cover a range of environments from declining inner-city areas, such as Camberwell and Salford, to relatively prosperous regional centres, such as Nottingham and Southampton. Aberdeen, Oxford and Worcester include rural areas as well. There is, however, no area whose predominant characteristic is social isolation, a factor that is likely to be related to high rates of suicide, and conditions such as schizophrenia that are associated with an increased risk of dependence and need for long-term care.

The factors that need to be taken into account when comparing register statistics can be classified under three headings: population dynamics, socio-demographic indices, and trends in policy. Detailed tables are provided in the appendices to Gibbons *et al* (1984).

Population dynamics

The population trends between 1921 and 1981, taken from census data for the seven register areas in England and Wales, are summarised in Fig. 1 and, for 1976–83, in Table 1. There are three clear groups: Oxford and Worcester attracted large numbers of people from elsewhere in the country; Cardiff, Nottingham and Southampton increased in population in line with the national trends; and Salford and Camberwell steadily decreased in size. The differences are remarkable. In Oxford, the population more than doubled in 60 years, while that of Camberwell decreased by half. Aberdeen is not shown in Fig. 1, but its population was steady until 1971, since when there has been an increase, due mainly to the expansion of the oil industry.

It is highly likely, therefore, that there has been a loss of aspirant groups from Camberwell, and to a lesser extent from Salford, over many decades, and a concomitant recruitment to places like Oxford and Worcester. (The population of Camberwell, which increased rapidly during the Industrial Revolution, reached its peak in 1911.) Population movement on such a scale must have been differentially associated with changes in the socio-demographic structure of the areas concerned.

Socio-demographic indices

There are only slight differences in age structure between register areas, and they all show the effects of the dramatic nationwide increase in the numbers of people over 65 years of age.

Social indicators show that register areas can be divided into decaying inner-city areas (Camberwell and Salford), medium-sized commercial and industrial cities (Cardiff, Nottingham and Southampton), and prosperous areas of population growth (Oxford and Worcester). Each, of course, has its own variability – the Oxford area is not uniformly attractive and Camberwell includes Dulwich Village (see Wing *et al* (1972) for an analysis of Camberwell wards). Oxford and Worcester stand out as being relatively privileged on several indicators (e.g. better housing conditions, fewer single parents). Camberwell stands out as being markedly underprivileged on almost every indicator. According to the recently introduced Jarman (1983) index of deprivation, the Camberwell health district is the seventh most deprived in England. Salford is similar to Camberwell in many respects, but in others comes closer to the intermediate group of industrial and commercial cities.

Government economic activity tables also show that Worcester and Oxford are the most privileged, but the differences between areas are not as clear cut as those discussed above, and Salford is less favoured than Camberwell in these respects. Aberdeen is more privileged than Scotland as a whole. Compared with England and Wales it is approximately at the average, in some respects a little better off than the industrial cities, in others a little less so.

Local policies, services and traditions

The third factor to be taken into account in explaining current differences in register statistics is historical. The services in Nottingham, for example, are still to some extent influenced by policies adopted during the 1950s and 1960s by a distinguished and effective psychiatrist, Dr Duncan Macmillan (Brown *et al*, 1966; Wing & Brown, 1970). The history of the Bethlem Royal and Maudsley joint hospital is, of course, unique, and Camberwell services have changed radically since this part of the borough of Southwark was taken over in 1967.

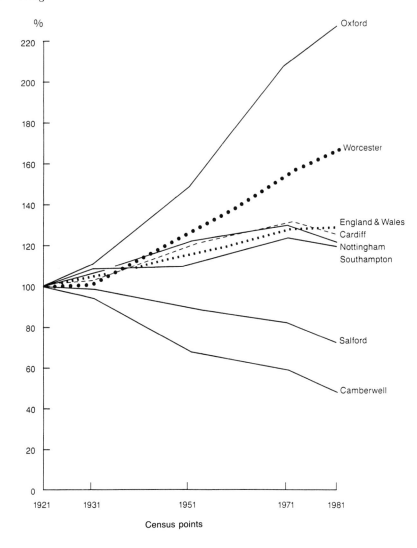

Fig. 1. Percentage population change, 1921–81 (1921 = 100%)

Oxford is unique in a different way. Worcester was singled out for special development in order to provide a model of the service described in "Better Services for the Mentally Ill" (DHSS, 1975). The pattern of services in every register area has been formed by myriad influences, only some of which can now be traced and recorded. Some of the local characteristics relevant to specific topics are described in later chapters.

Plan of the book

In Part II of the book, register statistics are described and considered. Chapter 2 contains an expanded series of tables relating to in-patient services. In the

TABLE 1
Estimated population size in register areas, 1976–83[1]

	1976	1977	1978	1979	1980	1981	1982	1983
All ages								
Camberwell	138 767	136 163	133 560	130 956	128 353	125 749	123 146	120 542
Salford	261 880	258 278	254 676	251 074	247 472	243 870	240 268	236 666
Southampton	210 229	209 250	208 272	207 294	206 315	205 337	204 359	203 380
Nottingham	394 354	391 487	388 621	385 755	382 889	380 023	377 157	374 291
Cardiff	—	279 155	277 748	276 340	274 933	273 525	272 117	270 708
Worcester	315 581	318 022	320 463	322 905	325 346	327 787	330 228	332 669
Oxford	482 309	486 382	490 456	494 530	498 603	502 677	506 751	510 824
Aberdeen	501 237	506 385	411 534	516 831	526 979	532 127	537 276	
Edinburgh	445 260	443 595	441 930	440 266	438 601	436 936	435 271	433 606
15–64 years								
Camberwell	90 893	89 488	88 084	86 680	85 274	83 869	82 464	81 058
Salford	165 397	163 462	161 526	159 592	157 657	155 722	153 787	151 852
Southampton	135 690	135 297	134 904	134 511	134 118	133 725	133 332	132 939
Nottingham	250 322	249 403	248 483	247 564	246 645	245 725	244 806	243 886
Cardiff	—	178 521	178 163	177 804	177 446	177 088	176 730	176 372
Worcester	200 522	202 425	204 328	206 321	208 135	210 038	211 941	213 044
Oxford	316 400	320 700	325 000	329 300	333 600	338 000	342 300	346 600
Aberdeen	308 000	311 784	315 564	319 347	323 127	326 910	330 692	334 474
Edinburgh	285 543	284 231	282 920	281 609	280 298	278 987	277 676	276 365
65 years and over								
Camberwell	19 215	19 150	19 083	19 016	18 950	18 883	18 816	18 750
Salford	36 893	37 201	37 510	37 819	38 130	38 439	38 748	39 057
Southampton	29 119	29 493	29 869	30 243	30 617	30 992	31 367	31 741
Nottingham	52 636	53 198	53 760	54 322	54 884	55 446	56 008	56 570
Cardiff	—	40 046	40 411	40 777	41 142	41 507	41 872	42 238
Worcester	44 145	45 072	45 999	46 926	47 853	48 780	49 707	50 634
Oxford	57 500	58 800	60 100	61 500	62 900	64 200	65 500	66 900
Aberdeen	69 702	70 528	71 351	72 175	72 998	73 822	74 646	75 470
Edinburgh	68 246	68 801	69 357	69 912	70 468	71 023	71 579	72 134

1. The population figures from 1977 to 1980 were based on straight-line interpolation between the populations as recorded by the 1971 and 1981 censuses. The 1982 and 1983 figures were straight-line extrapolations of the 1971–81 trend.

light of the population changes and the socio-demographic information provided above, the service indices can be examined for likely correlations. Chapter 3 provides a summary of trends in the register statistics for one particular district, Salford, and places them into the context of local service. Chapter 4 shows the effect of correcting for population decline on the rates of long-term bed occupancy estimated from data from the Camberwell register. Some comment is also made on the possible effect of socio-economic differences and earlier policies. Chapter 5 is concerned with the 'run-down' of Powick Hospital, which used to serve what became the Worcester Development Area. It provides useful background information for the research projects now being concluded that will try to answer some pertinent questions as to whether, at least in an area with these characteristics, the new pattern of services is as acceptable and as effective as the old – or perhaps better.

Part III of the book deals with a number of specific topics, each of which raises basic questions about the nature of the services involved. The description in Chapter 6, for example, of differences in organisation of the community psychiatric nursing services, suggests that there may be disadvantages in too free an 'attachment' to general practice, unless a change in priority from the more to the less severely disabled is contemplated. Chapter 7 records differences in practice with respect to the elderly. Southampton is particularly well known for its programme of 'domiciliary' visiting. (The quotation marks are necessary because the financial implications are quite different from those associated with the common use of the term.) Chapter 8 provides some confirmation for earlier studies suggesting that interventions following attempted suicide are not associated with dramatic improvements in outcome.

Finally, in Part IV, the future of psychiatric registers is considered. Dr Sineke ten Horn, who runs the Groningen register with Professor Robert Giel, reports in Chapter 9 the extraordinary growth of registers in other parts of Europe. In many cases, the registers were based on UK models, but they are learning from each other and adapting, as our registers have had to do, to local pressures. We may confidently look forward to the first all-Europe volume of register studies.

The Department of Health has, in the past, given solid support to the establishment of case registers in the UK. It was particularly disappointing, therefore, that central funding was withdrawn from three registers at the end of March 1987. Chapter 10, by a civil servant with a long – in fact almost unique – experience of the administrative problems of mental health services, gives characteristically muted, but nonetheless explicit, expression to expectations that were, and perhaps still are, held in the Department.

This is followed, in Chapter 11, by what is, in effect, a challenge, both to the Department, which was responsible for endorsing the proposals of the Körner committee (1982), and to case registers, which have the potential, if not always the resources, to undertake something more imaginative, far reaching and useful. The limitations of the Körner proposals, and the problems likely to be encountered in their execution, are explained by Professor Cooper, who summarises the experience of all the registers. In the final chapter, some of these matters are reconsidered and the opportunities available to registers through rapid advances in computer technology are explored. The term 'expert system' has become a cliché or, worse, a gimmick. But, properly used, computers can provide professional caring staff with means for immensely improving the quality of their practice, and district planners with a medicosocial information system that provides a rich and realistic database for 'bottom-up' planning.

References

BAHN, A. K., GARDNER, E. A., ALLTOP, L., *et al* (1966) Comparative study of rates of admission and prevalence for psychiatric facilities in four register areas. *American Journal of Public Health*, **56**, 2033.

BROWN, G. W., BONE, M., DALISON, B., *et al* (1966) *Schizophrenia and Social Care*. London: Oxford University Press.

DEPARTMENT OF HEALTH AND SOCIAL SECURITY (1974) Proceedings of psychiatric case register conference, Aberdeen. *DHSS Statistical Report Series No. 13*. London: HMSO.

—— (1975) *Better Services for the Mentally Ill.* Command 6233. London: HMSO.

GIBBONS, J., JENNINGS, C. & WING, J. K. (1984) *Psychiatric Care in Eight Register Areas.* Southampton: University Department of Psychiatry. (Copies obtainable by sending £2.50, cheque payable to University of Southampton, to University Department of Psychiatry, Royal South Hants Hospital, Southampton SO9 4PE.)

JARMAN, B. (1983) Identification of underprivileged areas. *British Medical Journal,* **286,** 1705–1709.

WING, J. K. & BRANSBY, R. (1970) Psychiatric case registers. *DHSS Statistical Report Series No. 8.* London: HMSO.

—— & BROWN, G. W. (1970) *Institutionalism and Schizophrenia.* London: Cambridge University Press.

—— & FRYERS, T. (1976) *Psychiatric Services in Camberwell and Salford: Statistics from the Camberwell and Salford Psychiatric Registers* (mimeo). Salford: Salford Register.

WING, L., WING, J. K., HAILEY, A., *et al* (1967) The use of psychiatric services in three urban areas: an international case register study. *Social Psychiatry,* **2,** 158–167.

——, BALDWIN, J. A. & ROSEN, B. M. (1972) The use of child psychiatric services in three urban areas: an international case register study. In *Evaluating a Community Psychiatric Service: The Camberwell Register 1964–71* (eds J. K. Wing & A. M. Hailey), pp. 101–114. London: Oxford University Press.

II. Statistics

2 In-patient statistics from eight psychiatric case registers, 1977-83

C. JENNINGS, G. DER, C. ROBINSON, S. ROSE, J. DE ALARCON, D. HUNTER, R. HOLLIDAY and N. MOSS

This chapter presents statistics showing the level, variation and dynamics of in-patient care in eight areas of Britain covered by case registers. The statistics update and extend the in-patient tables in our previous comparative case register report *Psychiatric Care in 8 Register Areas* (Gibbons *et al*, 1984).

The chapter covers admission rates, their trends, relation to national figures, and variation by age and diagnosis. The length of stay of those who are discharged or die is also included. The resident in-patient statistics cover rates, trends, composition by length of stay and comparisons with national rates. The composition and dynamics of the long-stay groups are explored by tables showing the age and diagnosis of long-stay patients and the proportions joining, leaving and staying in the medium-long-stay and very-long-stay groups. This last analysis should be of interest to those concerned with predicting the build up and run down of numbers of long-stay psychiatric in-patients. Two other questions are examined: the extent to which the elderly very-long-stay group are those admitted before age 65 who have become old in hospital, and the difference that changing to a more clinically relevant definition of length of stay makes to its distribution.

Three detailed tables cover the period 1977 to 1983 and most trend comparisons within the text compare 1977 with 1983. Almost all the tables are divided into the age groups 15-64 and 65 and over. The two age groups are very different clinically and this is reflected in the rates and the trends in the rates reported here.

Admissions and discharges

This section covers admission rates by year, age, and clinical group, together with discharges and deaths by length of stay, year and age. Admissions include all events initiating a spell of psychiatric in-patient care, and so include, for example, transfers from a non-psychiatric general hospital. Readmissions to hospital have been counted as admissions no matter how short the time since the last discharge. Transfers from one psychiatric hospital to another within the area covered by the register have been ignored; such transfers have not been counted in either the admission or discharge tables and the length of stay has been calculated from the original admission.

Table 2 summarises admission rates by year and age group for 1977-83 for each register area, and this information is given in detail in Table 3.

TABLE 2
Admission rates per 100 000 population, 1983, by age group, and percentage difference 1977–83

15–64			65 and over			15 and over		
	Rate	% differ-ence 1977–83		Rate	% differ-ence 1977–83		Rates	% differ-ence 1977–83
Southampton	578	+ 4	Southampton	1881	+ 20	Southampton	671	+ 13
Camberwell	567	+ 10				Camberwell	506	– 9
All Scotland	537	– 11	All Scotland	1056	+ 38	All Scotland	502	+ 5
Edinburgh	508	– 11	Edinburgh	1047	+ 30	Edinburgh	498	+ 1
Aberdeen	491	– 12	Worcester	1045	+ 92	Cardiff[1]	469	+ 3
Cardiff[1]	481	+ 10	Oxford	990	+ 40	Salford	442	+ 20
Salford	463	+ 2	Cardiff[1]	977	– 17	Aberdeen	431	– 2
			Aberdeen	890	+ 29	Worcester	420	+ 50
			Salford	881	+ 52			
All England	418	– 7	All England	830	+ 37	All England	398	+ 6
Worcester	405	+ 27	Camberwell	800	– 21	Oxford	385	– 3
Oxford	377	– 20						

1. Cardiff, 1978–83.

Table 2 shows admission rates per 100 000 total population, by age group. For all those aged 15 and over, Southampton had the highest rate, nearly 70% above the rate for all of England. The other areas, except Oxford, had rates above the national rate, but within 30% of it. Nationally the admission rate increased 6% over the period 1977–83. In five register areas the rate increased, in Salford and Worcester by substantial amounts. In the younger age group, most register areas had higher rates than England as a whole (11–38% higher). The rates for Worcester and Oxford were slightly lower than the national rate, while the highest rates occurred in Southampton and Camberwell. Between 1977 and 1983, admission rates in England, the Scottish areas and Oxford fell, while the other areas showed modest rises of up to 10%, except in Worcester where there was a rise of a quarter. In the elderly age group, most areas had a higher rate than England as a whole, the excess ranging from 6% to 26%, except in Southampton where the rate was nearly 1900, more than twice as high as the England rate. The rate for Camberwell, in contrast to the younger age group, was lower than the England rate. Nationally the admission rate for the elderly increased by nearly 40% between 1977 and 1983. Substantial increases of 20–90% were noted in all register areas except Cardiff and Camberwell where rates fell by about 20%. In Worcester a substantial part of the increase occurred in 1983 after a consultant psychogeriatrician had been appointed.

In 1983, age-specific admission rates for the elderly were much higher than the rates for those aged 15–64. A ratio of 2:1 applied in four register areas and for all England; in Worcester and Oxford the ratio was higher (2.6:1), owing to a lower than average rate in the 15–64 age group; in Camberwell the ratio was only 1.4:1, owing to the low rate for the elderly.

Do differences in admission rates actually reflect differences in the number of people admitted, or do they merely reflect policy (for example, the use of repeated short admissions)? To test this we calculated rates for persons admitted during a year and the ratio of admissions to persons admitted. If the ratio of admissions to persons admitted was highest in areas with high admission rates,

TABLE 3

In-patient admission rates per 100 000 population by year and age group, 1977–83

	1977	1978	1979	1980	1981	1982	1983
15 years and over: rates in total population							
Camberwell	558	547	532	593	564	486	506
Salford	373	373	340	393	404	382	442
Southampton	596	585	575	647	705	691	671
Cardiff	—	454	447	463	446	422	469
Worcester	280	293	343	355	337	368	420
Oxford	396	376	416	429	439	435	385
England	374	367	361	383	392	388	398
Wales (16–64)	399	405	400	423	427	423	449
Aberdeen	442	449	459	481	482	418	431
Edinburgh	493	502	489	476	450	451	498
Scotland	480	477	475	496	502	452	501
15–65 years: age-specific rates							
Camberwell	631	605	576	640	626	564	567
Salford	456	429	397	452	442	399	463
Southampton	556	526	493	527	622	594	578
Cardiff	—	437	438	465	442	418	481
Worcester	319	304	355	386	354	375	405
Oxford	470	443	461	464	471	446	377
England	451	431	416	431	433	416	418
Wales (16–64)	493	476	459	487	483	464	484
Aberdeen	562	574	573	575	555	478	491
Edinburgh	574	573	567	528	541	480	508
Scotland	597	578	565	580	570	497	537
65 years and over: age-specific rates							
Camberwell	1018	1038	1041	1135	974	707	800
Salford	581	685	579	682	773	777	881
Southampton	1682	1704	1746	2051	1984	1977	1881
Cardiff	—	1195	1123	1086	1058	979	997
Worcester	544	691	797	738	738	847	1045
Oxford	707	671	876	940	953	1037	990
England	608	629	639	712	743	770	830
Wales	648	739	764	785	811	845	921
Aberdeen	691	681	748	889	986	861	890
Edinburgh	807	862	797	863	784	883	1047
Scotland	767	810	826	887	955	904	1056

it would suggest that the use of repeated short admissions was affecting admission rates. We found little evidence that this was the case. In the younger age group, admission rates were around 30% higher than rates for persons admitted, except in Southampton and Oxford where admission rates were 40–50% higher in some years. Since Oxford admission rates were low, it is only in Southampton that part, but only part, of the high admission rate could be a result of higher rates of readmissions. In the older age group, ratios of admissions to persons admitted varied quite widely (from 1.2 to 2.0) but, on the whole, areas with high admission rates also had high rates for persons admitted, so repeated short admissions are not an explanation for this variation. They may, however, need to be taken into account in explaining the absolute level in some areas.

Tables 4 and 5 show 1983 admission rates per 100 000 for each area, and the percentage distributions of the major clinical groups, by age group. In the

TABLE 4

In-patient admission rates and percentage distribution of the major clinical groups[1] (in parentheses) by age group, 1983

	15–64 years				65 years and over		
	SP	AF	AD	OT	DM	AF	OT
Age-specific rates							
Camberwell	189 (33)	211 (37)	67 (12)	100 (18)	309 (39)	224 (28)	267 (33)
Southampton	159 (28)	218 (38)	93 (16)	108 (19)	816 (43)	772 (41)	293 (16)
Cardiff	133 (28)	165 (34)	75 (16)	108 (22)	462 (46)	285 (27)	250 (27)
Salford	124 (27)	147 (32)	72 (16)	120 (26)	269 (31)	292 (33)	317 (36)
Edinburgh	110 (22)	166 (33)	122 (24)	110 (22)	606 (58)	281 (27)	160 (15)
Worcester	87 (21)	153 (38)	62 (15)	104 (26)	533 (51)	320 (31)	192 (18)
Aberdeen	72 (15)	198 (40)	120 (24)	101 (20)	416 (47)	343 (39)	131 (15)
Oxford	57 (15)	86 (23)	144 (39)	84 (23)	584 (59)	201 (20)	203 (20)
Rates per 100 000 total population							
Camberwell	127 (33)	142 (37)	45 (12)	68 (18)	48 (39)	35 (28)	41 (33)
Southampton	104 (28)	142 (38)	61 (16)	70 (19)	127 (43)	120 (41)	46 (16)
Cardiff	87 (28)	107 (34)	49 (16)	71 (22)	72 (46)	41 (27)	42 (27)
Salford	80 (27)	94 (32)	46 (16)	76 (26)	44 (31)	48 (33)	52 (36)
Edinburgh	70 (22)	106 (33)	77 (24)	70 (22)	101 (58)	47 (27)	27 (15)
Worcester	56 (21)	99 (38)	40 (15)	67 (26)	81 (51)	49 (31)	29 (18)
Aberdeen	45 (15)	123 (40)	75 (24)	63 (20)	58 (47)	48 (39)	18 (15)
Oxford	39 (15)	59 (23)	99 (39)	59 (23)	77 (59)	26 (20)	26 (20)

1. See footnote to Table 5.

TABLE 5

In-patient admission rates, per 100 000 total population, and percentage distribution of the major clinical groups[1] (in parentheses), patients aged 15 and over, 1983

	SP	AF	AD	DM	OT
Camberwell	145 (29)	177 (35)	46 (9)	50 (10)	88 (17)
Southampton	117 (17)	263 (39)	62 (9)	133 (20)	97 (15)
Cardiff	95 (20)	149 (32)	53 (11)	76 (16)	96 (20)
Salford	96 (22)	142 (32)	49 (11)	46 (10)	109 (25)
Edinburgh	80 (16)	153 (31)	83 (17)	104 (21)	78 (16)
Worcester	63 (15)	147 (35)	44 (11)	87 (21)	78 (19)
Aberdeen	51 (12)	172 (40)	79 (18)	61 (14)	68 (16)
Oxford	49 (13)	86 (22)	102 (26)	78 (20)	73 (19)

1. SP = Schizophrenic and paranoid psychoses (Group 1)
   AF = Affective psychoses and neuroses   (Groups 2 and 3)
   AD = Alcohol- and drug-related disorders (Group 4)
   DM = Dementia   (Group 6)
   OT = Other disorders   (Groups 5, 7, 8 and 9)
   ICD–9 codes (World Health Organization, 1978):
   Group 1. Schizophrenia and paranoid psychoses (295 Schizophrenic psychoses, 297 Paranoid states, 298.3 Acute paranoid reaction, 298.4 Psychogenic paranoid psychosis)
   Group 2. Affective psychoses (296 Affective psychoses, 298.0 Other non-organic psychoses, depressed type, 298.1 Other non-organic psychoses, excitative type)
   Group 3. Other depression (300.4 Neurotic depression, 309.0 Brief depressive reaction, 209.1 Prolonged depressive reaction, 311 Depressive disorder, not elsewhere classified)
   Group 4. Alcohol- and drug-related disorders (291 Alcoholic psychoses, 292 Drug psychoses, 303 Alcohol dependence syndrome, 304 Drug dependence, 305 Non-dependent abuse of drugs)
   Group 5. Other neurosis (excluding neurotic depression) (300 Neurotic disorders (except 300.4))
   Group 6. Dementia (290 Senile and presenile organic psychotic conditions)
   Group 7. Other organic disorders (293 Transient organic psychotic conditions, 294 Other organic psychotic conditions (chronic), 310 Specific non-psychotic mental disorder following organic brain damage)
   Group 8. Personality disorders (301 Personality disorders)
   Group 9. Other (298.2 Reactive confusion, 298.8 Other and unspecified reactive psychosis, 298.9 Unspecified psychosis, 299 Psychoses with origin specific to childhood, 302 Sexual deviations and disorders, 306 Physiological malfunction arising from mental factors, 307 Special symptoms or syndromes not elsewhere classified, 308 Acute reaction to stress, 309 Adjustment reaction (except 309.0, 309.1), 312 Disturbance of conduct not elsewhere classified, 313 Disturbance of emotions specific to childhood and adolescence, 314 Hyperkinetic syndrome of childhood, 315 Specific delays in development, 316 Psychic factors associated with diseases classified elsewhere, 317–319 Mental retardation).

younger age group around a third of admissions were given a diagnosis of affective psychosis or other depressive disorder ('AF'), and rates ranged from 150 to 220, except in Oxford, where only a quarter of patients were in this category and the rate was only 86. The 'OT' category, which included non-depressive neurosis and personality disorders among other conditions, accounted for around 20% of admissions in most areas, with a rate of 100–120, except in Oxford where the rate was again lower. Admissions for alcohol- and drug-related conditions ('AD') occurred at a rate of 60–90 in five areas, accounting for around 15% of admissions. In Oxford and the Scottish areas, however, the rates were much higher, at 120–150. In Scotland around a quarter of admissions were in this group, while in Oxford 40% of admissions were for alcohol- or drug-related conditions. The widest variation however was in the schizophrenia and paranoid states group ('SP'), with rates of 189 in Camberwell and 57 in Oxford – more than a threefold range. The proportion of admissions in this category ranged from 15% to 33%.

In the older age group, the differences between areas were in large measure due to variation in rates for dementia ('DM'). In the depressive category ('AF'), rates ranged from 200 to 340, except in Southampton where the rate was nearly 800. The percentage of admissions in the depressive category ranged from 20% to 40%. The 'OT' category was rather more widely spread, with rates from 130 to 320. Rates for dementia, however, varied over a threefold range, from 270 to 820, although the highest rate, in Southampton, was exceptional, the next highest rate being 600 in Edinburgh. Similarly the percentage of admissions with dementia varied between 30% and 60%. Southampton had extremely high elderly admission rates because of the deliberate policy of the psychogeriatricians, and these admissions were fairly evenly split between those with dementia and those who were depressed.

Tables 6 and 7 are concerned with the length of stay of those discharged from or dying in in-patient care. Table 6 shows median lengths of stay. A typical figure for the younger age group in 1983 was 19 days, although in Southampton and Oxford the median stay was almost half this figure, while in Camberwell it was more than twice as much. In Southampton, Oxford and, to a lesser extent, Cardiff, the median length of stay declined substantially after 1977, while in the other areas it changed only slightly, usually increasing. Median lengths of stay for the elderly were higher than in the younger age group and more variable, ranging in 1983 from 14 days in Oxford up to 89 days in Camberwell. The trend between 1977 and 1983 was downward in five areas and slightly upward in two areas, while in Camberwell there was a substantial rise.

Table 7 shows in-patient discharges and deaths in 1983 by age and time spent in hospital. From 10% to 20% of all those discharged or dying had lengths of stay of less than one week, except for Oxford, with 27%, a reflection perhaps of the large proportion of admissions with alcohol-related problems. However, the elderly were much less likely than those under 65 to be discharged within a week. The proportion of elderly patients who had stayed less than a week was 5–10% compared with a typical 20% in the younger age group (although in Southampton and Oxford around a third were discharged within a week). In most areas except Camberwell, between two-thirds and three-quarters of the discharges and deaths followed lengths of stay of less than one month. There was less difference between the age groups, although in everywhere except

TABLE 6

Median[1] length of stay of patients discharged from or dying in in-patient care, 1977 and 1983, by age

	15–64		65 and over		15 and over	
	1977	*1983*	*1977*	*1983*	*1977*	*1983*
Camberwell	41	43	70	88.5	48	48
Aberdeen	18.5	20.5	40.5	41.5	22.5	24
Cardiff[2]	22.5[3]	19.4[3]	23.3[3]	25.6[3]	22.9[3]	22[3]
Salford	19.6[3]	19.7[3]	40[3]	37[3]	21	21.5
Worcester	18.5[3]	19.1[3]	29.5[3]	25[3]	21.4[3]	21.3[3]
Edinburgh	20	18	40	23	24	20
Southampton	17	12	23	19.5	20	15
Oxford	15	10	20	14	17	14

1. The medians were calculated using the exact number of days in hospital except in Cardiff, Worcester and Salford where they were estimated from the grouped length-of-stay distribution. The length-of-stay categories used were (in days): 0–6, 7–13, 14–30, 31–60, 61–182, 183–364, 365–1825, 1826 and over. Comparisons in other areas showed group estimation usually produced medians 2–3 days greater than that produced by the exact method where the median lay between 14 and 30 days. The difference was greater when the median exceeded 30 days.
2. Cardiff, 1978–83.
3. Median estimated from grouped data.

TABLE 7

Percentage of in-patients discharged or dying in 1983, by length of stay

	Less than 1 week			Less than 1 month			Less than 6 months		
	15–64	*65 and over*	*15 and over*	*15–64*	*65 and over*	*15 and over*	*15–64*	*65 and over*	*15 and over*
Camberwell	11	6	10	38	24	35	90	68	85
Aberdeen	16	5	13	63	32	54	93	68	86
Edinburgh	19	7	15	67	58	64	95	87	92
Worcester	20	10	16	74	60	69	98	89	95
Salford	22	7	17	69	46	61	95	80	89
Cardiff	25	10	20	66	60	64	96	84	92
Southampton	34	6	21	79	70	75	97	95	96
Oxford	37	9	27	73	73	73	97	91	95

Oxford more of the younger age group had been discharged within the month. At least 85% and in most cases over 90% of the discharges followed a stay of less than six months, leaving as few as 5% discharged after stays of more than six months.

Resident in-patients

The count of resident in-patients includes all those in hospital on 31 December. In this section, we discuss the differences between register areas and the trends over 1977–83 for each length-of-stay group. Three main groups are considered: the short-stay patients who had been in hospital for less than a year, the medium-long-stay, who had been in hospital for between one and five years, and the very-long-stay, who had been in hospital for more than five years. Within the medium-long and very-long-stay groups special attention is paid to the numbers joining these groups or leaving through discharge or death. There are also analyses of the age at admission of very-long-stay elderly patients, age and clinical distributions of long-stay (more than one year) patients, and a study of the effect of changing the method of calculating length of stay. Detailed figures are

TABLE 8

Numbers of discharges and deaths of those (aged 15 and over) in hospital at the previous 31 December, by length of stay, 1977–83[1]

	1977	1978	1979	1980	1981	1982	1983
Camberwell							
1 year	137	143	133	108	144	112	111
1–5 years	20	25	20	24	24	21	25
5 years and over	10	18	15	17	16	20	10
Total	163	186	168	149	184	153	146
Salford							
1 year	93	92	86	88	94	105	97
1–5 years	14	17	28	30	30	36	34
5 years and over	30	29	20	32	32	25	37
Total	137	138	134	150	156	166	168
Southampton							
1 year	133	116	112	101	110	123	94
1–5 years	21	24	20	20	19	14	17
5 years and over	20	14	9	10	14	10	9
Total	174	154	141	131	143	147	120
Cardiff							
1 year	–	113	135	134	119	138	132
1–5 years	–	37	43	32	35	29	38
5 years and over	–	18	30	21	23	26	23
Total	–	168	208	187	177	193	193
Worcester							
1 year	72	76	89	105	94	113	112
1–5 years	21	28	21	21	25	14	26
5 years and over	28	27	35	21	16	16	19
Total	121	131	145	147	135	143	157
Oxford							
1 year	158	163	165	146	163	152	164
1–5 years	36	26	39	35	32	29	28
5 years and over	21	17	20	19	23	14	10
Total	215	206	224	200	218	195	202

1. Age and length of stay as at previous 31 December.

given in Tables 8 and 9. In all the tables except Table 20 the 'continuous-stay' method of calculating length of stay has been used. The definition given under 'Admissions and discharges' (above) was used to determine what should be counted as an admission and therefore when the starting point for calculating duration of stay should be. This means that if a patient left the psychiatric hospital for a short period, whether discharged to the community or (say) going to a general hospital for an operation, that would count as a break in care and the length of stay would be calculated from the date on which he returned to the psychiatric hospital. This tends to shorten lengths of stay.

National figures for England, Wales and Scotland have been included, and some comparisons are made. It should be noted that the national figures count transfers between hospitals as new admissions, whereas the register figures ignore transfers between local hospitals. The result of this is that national figures will slightly underestimate the number of longer-stay patients and overestimate the number of short-stay patients compared with registers. The basis for estimation of the number of resident in-patients in England was changed from 1980.

TABLE 9

Resident in-patients, 31 December 1977 to 1983, by length of stay and age group – rates per 100 000 total population

Length of stay by district	15–64 years							65 years and over							15 years and over						
	1977	1978	1979	1980	1981	1982	1983	1977	1978	1979	1980	1981	1982	1983	1977	1978	1979	1980	1981	1982	1983
Camberwell																					
<1 year	69.8	76.4	68.7	77.9	66.8	77.1	71.3	55.1	42.7	39.7	60.0	47.7	30.9	39.8	124.9	119.0	108.4	137.9	114.5	108.0	111.2
1–2 years	10.3	5.2	12.2	12.5	8.0	13.0	9.1	10.3	15.7	7.6	11.7	16.7	16.2	10.0	20.6	21.0	19.9	24.2	24.7	29.2	19.1
2–5 years	7.3	9.0	10.7	14.8	8.0	9.7	14.9	22.0	18.7	19.1	11.7	17.5	20.3	23.2	29.4	27.7	29.8	26.5	25.4	30.0	38.2
5–6 years	2.2	1.5	1.5	0.8	5.6	0.8	0.8	4.4	3.0	3.8	3.9	1.6	3.2	0.8	6.6	4.5	5.3	4.7	7.2	4.1	1.7
6 years and over	40.4	36.7	35.1	32.7	25.4	25.2	24.1	63.2	61.4	58.0	54.5	55.7	49.5	46.5	103.6	98.1	93.2	87.3	81.1	74.7	70.5
Total	130	129	128	139	114	126	120	155	142	128	142	139	120	120	285.0	270.3	256.6	280.5	252.9	246.0	240.6
1–5 years	18	14	23	27	16	23	24	32	34	27	23	34	37	33	49.9	48.7	49.6	50.6	50.1	59.3	57.2
5 years and over	43	38	37	34	31	26	25	68	64	62	58	57	53	47	110.2	102.6	98.5	91.9	88.3	78.8	72.2
Salford																					
<1 year	27.1	25.1	34.3	25.9	32.8	30.0	35.1	25.2	29.1	25.9	28.3	36.1	31.2	28.7	52.3	54.2	60.1	54.1	68.9	61.2	63.8
1–2 years	10.1	5.9	6.8	8.1	6.2	8.7	9.7	11.6	11.0	14.3	16.2	10.3	17.9	13.9	21.7	16.9	20.7	24.2	16.4	26.6	23.7
2–5 years	11.2	16.5	14.3	13.3	11.5	9.6	11.8	17.8	23.2	24.7	26.7	30.3	25.8	30.0	27.1	39.7	39.0	40.0	41.8	35.4	41.8
5–6 years	2.7	1.6	2.0	2.8	5.7	2.5	1.3	3.1	3.9	5.2	5.7	5.7	6.2	5.1	5.8	5.5	7.2	8.5	11.5	8.7	6.3
6 years and over	54.6	51.4	48.6	43.6	40.2	42.0	40.1	54.2	53.4	55.4	56.2	58.2	58.7	55.4	108.8	104.8	104.0	99.8	98.4	100.7	95.5
Total	106	101	106	94	94	93	98	112	121	125	133	141	140	133	215.7	221.1	231.0	226.7	237.0	232.7	231.1
1–5 years	21	22	21	21	18	18	22	29	34	39	43	41	44	44	48.8	56.5	59.7	64.2	58.2	62.0	65.5
5 years and over	57	53	51	46	46	45	41	57	57	61	62	64	65	60	114.6	110.3	111.1	108.3	109.9	109.5	101.8
Southampton																					
<1 year	40.1	35.1	30.4	33.0	38.5	26.4	29.0	30.1	32.2	30.4	31.5	34.1	29.8	30.0	70.3	67.2	60.8	64.5	72.6	56.3	59.0
1–2 years	8.1	8.2	4.8	6.3	5.4	4.4	5.4	8.1	6.7	8.7	5.8	5.8	7.3	5.4	16.2	14.9	13.5	12.1	11.2	11.7	10.8
2–5 years	6.7	8.6	12.1	10.2	8.8	7.8	7.9	10.0	9.6	9.6	12.1	14.1	11.3	11.8	16.7	18.2	21.7	22.3	22.9	19.1	19.7
5–6 years	1.4	1.0	1.0	1.9	2.4	4.9	1.5	1.4	2.4	1.0	1.5	0.0	3.4	2.0	2.9	3.4	1.9	2.4	2.4	8.3	3.4
6 years and over	26.3	23.5	22.2	21.8	19.0	18.6	21.1	19.1	18.2	18.8	16.5	16.1	14.2	15.7	45.4	41.8	41.0	38.3	35.1	32.8	36.9
Total	83	76	70	73	74	62	65	69	69	69	67	70	66	65	151.5	145.5	138.9	140.6	144.2	128.2	129.8
1–5 years	15	17	17	16	14	12	13	18	16	18	18	20	19	17	33.0	33.1	35.2	34.3	34.1	30.8	30.5
5 years and over	28	24	23	24	21	23	23	21	21	20	18	16	18	18	48.3	45.1	42.9	41.7	37.5	41.1	40.3

TABLE 9 (continued)

Cardiff

Age group	1	2	3	4	5	6	7	8	9	10	11	12	13	14	15	16	17	18	19	20
<1 year	31.5	36.7	36.2	29.1	38.8	32.3	33.2	27.6	32.9	29.5	27.8	30.1	29.6	59.1	64.1	69.1	58.6	66.5	62.5	62.8
1–2 years	3.6	7.2	5.1	6.2	4.0	5.9	4.1	11.5	10.5	14.5	12.4	10.3	10.0	15.0	18.7	15.6	20.7	16.5	16.2	14.0
2–5 years	11.5	7.6	9.0	8.4	9.5	3.5	8.5	32.6	24.6	20.4	21.2	20.2	17.7	44.1	38.2	33.7	28.7	30.7	28.7	26.2
5–6 years	2.1	2.9	2.5	1.5	1.1	2.6	1.5	3.2	5.1	7.6	4.0	4.0	3.0	5.4	7.9	7.6	9.1	5.1	6.6	4.4
6 years and over	34.4	32.4	27.9	27.3	24.9	22.0	23.3	27.6	30.8	31.5	34.7	34.5	31.8	62.0	61.6	58.6	58.6	59.6	56.6	55.0
Total	83	87	81	72	78	71	71	102	104	103	100	99	92	185.6	190.5	184.6	175.7	178.4	170.5	162.5
1–5 years	15	15	14	15	13	14	13	44	35	35	34	31	28	59.1	56.9	49.2	49.5	47.2	44.8	40.3
5 years and over	37	35	30	29	26	25	25	31	36	39	39	39	35	67.3	69.5	66.2	67.7	64.7	63.2	59.5

Worcester

Age group	1	2	3	4	5	6	7	8	9	10	11	12	13	14	15	16	17	18	19	20
<1 year	14.8	15.6	20.4	18.7	18.9	13.2	19.5	17.9	22.6	22.6	22.4	23.1	16.3	32.7	39.0	43.0	35.0	41.5	40.6	42.7
1–2 years	3.1	1.6	3.1	1.8	1.5	0.6	0.9	6.9	7.1	4.9	6.7	6.0	6.8	10.1	9.7	10.2	8.6	3.4	7.3	6.9
2–5 years	7.2	5.3	4.0	4.9	4.0	3.9	1.2	11.9	10.2	9.8	8.5	7.2	11.1	19.2	15.0	14.2	16.0	13.7	12.4	8.4
5–6 years	0.9	2.8	1.2	0.3	1.5	0.9	1.2	3.8	0.9	1.8	1.8	2.4	1.5	4.7	5.9	2.2	1.8	3.4	2.7	3.6
6 years and over	23.3	20.9	20.7	19.1	16.8	16.7	16.2	50.6	42.1	37.8	35.4	31.9	39.0	73.9	69.3	62.9	58.1	24.1	52.1	48.1
Total	49	46	50	45	43	40	39	91	83	77	75	71	75	140.6	138.9	132.5	119.6	116.5	115.1	109.7
1–5 years	10	7	7	7	5	5	2	19	17	15	15	13	18	29.2	24.7	24.5	24.6	17.1	19.7	15.3
5 years and over	24	24	22	19	18	18	17	54	43	40	37	34	41	78.6	75.2	65.0	59.9	58.0	54.8	51.7

Oxford

Age group	1	2	3	4	5	6	7	8	9	10	11	12	13	14	15	16	17	18	19	20
<1 year	29.6	27.5	21.0	25.7	21.1	22.7	20.8	13.2	16.6	13.5	16.1	16.6	13.8	42.8	41.0	37.6	39.5	37.2	39.7	37.4
1–2 years	4.3	4.3	3.2	1.8	1.8	2.2	2.2	4.1	4.0	4.9	5.0	4.7	6.2	8.4	9.2	7.3	8.0	6.8	6.9	7.2
2–5 years	4.3	4.5	4.2	4.6	4.0	2.6	2.3	7.4	6.7	7.7	6.6	7.7	5.2	11.7	12.2	10.9	9.8	10.5	10.3	9.6
5–6 years	0.2	1.2	1.2	0.4	0.4	0.8	0.8	1.0	1.2	1.2	0.4	0.4	0.8	1.2	2.4	2.2	1.2	0.8	1.2	2.0
6 years and over	9.5	8.4	8.1	6.6	6.0	5.3	5.7	18.7	15.8	17.3	12.7	11.2	15.6	28.2	25.7	23.9	22.3	18.7	16.2	15.7
Total	48	46	38	39	33	34	32	44	44	45	41	41	42	92.3	90.5	81.9	80.8	74.0	74.6	71.8
1–5 years	9	9	7	6	6	5	5	12	11	13	12	12	11	20.1	21.4	18.2	17.8	17.3	17.2	16.8
5 years and over	10	10	9	7	6	6	6	20	17	19	13	12	16	29.4	28.1	26.1	23.5	19.5	17.8	17.6

Aberdeen

Age group	1	2	3	4	5	6	7	8	9	10	11	12	13	14	15	16	17	18	19	20	21
<1 year	43.4	48.9	45.9	43.5	50.5	44.9	40.9	31.4	33.8	34.3	33.8	40.6	52.0	46.0	74.8	82.7	80.1	84.1	102.5	91.0	90.8
1–2 years	11.7	8.4	11.4	9.0	9.3	14.5	10.6	17.8	17.4	19.9	17.1	19.9	20.5	25.3	29.4	25.8	31.4	26.1	29.8	46.0	35.9
2–5 years	19.4	20.3	14.9	13.8	10.6	12.8	17.1	34.4	34.6	33.9	30.9	25.0	30.4	38.9	53.7	54.9	48.8	44.7	35.7	43.2	56.0
5–6 years	3.0	3.9	4.8	2.1	4.2	1.7	3.5	5.7	6.3	5.6	6.5	6.3	6.3	5.2	8.7	10.2	10.5	8.6	8.6	5.1	8.7
6 years and over	44.8	40.1	37.7	36.8	34.3	33.5	31.3	64.4	62.9	61.2	56.3	56.3	52.9	45.2	109.2	103.0	98.9	93.1	87.3	84.0	76.5
Total	122	122	115	105	109	107	103	153	155	155	151	157	162	165	275.9	276.6	269.6	256.6	265.7	269.3	268.0
1–5 years	31	29	26	23	20	27	28	52	52	54	48	46	46	64	83.1	80.7	80.1	70.7	65.5	89.3	91.9
5 years and over	48	44	43	39	39	35	35	70	69	67	63	59	54	50	117.9	113.2	109.4	101.8	97.7	89.1	85.2

Until then the estimate was made by updating a 1971 census of psychiatric in-patients by adding admissions and subtracting discharges. From 1980 the estimate derived in this way has been scaled to make it agree with in-patient data given by age in the SBH 112 facilities return. The effect was to reduce the total number of patients in 1980 by about 1.5%, to increase the number aged 65 and over by a similar proportion, and to reduce the number aged 15–64 by 3–4%.

Table 10 shows resident in-patient rates on 31 December 1983 by length of stay and age. As in our previous report (Gibbons *et al*, 1984), the rates for English and Welsh areas for all resident in-patients fall into three groups. Camberwell and Salford had high rates, Southampton and Cardiff had rates similar to those for England as a whole, and Worcester and Oxford had low rates. Aberdeen had rates somewhat higher than those of Camberwell and Salford but slightly lower than the rate for Scotland as a whole.

Short-stay (less than one year) patients include acute patients together with chronic patients who have been recently readmitted. In the 15–64 age group, rates were twice as high in Camberwell as in England and were high also in the Scottish areas. Salford, Southampton and Cardiff had rates similar to England and Wales at 30–35 per 100 000, while rates in Worcester and Oxford were only 20 per 100 000. In the over 65 age group there was less variation in rates. The Scottish areas had rates of 50 per 100 000 while that for Camberwell was 40 per 100 000, much lower than in the younger age group. Salford, Southampton and Cardiff at 30 per 100 000 were just above the rates for England and Wales, while in Worcester and Oxford the rates were again lower, although in Worcester it was only 15% lower than the rate for England.

In the younger age group medium-long-stay rates in Camberwell, Salford, Aberdeen and all Scotland, at around 24 per 100 000, were twice as high as the rates for England. In Southampton and Cardiff rates were similar to the English rate, while in Worcester and Oxford rates were very low (2 and 5 per 100 000 respectively). In the elderly age group, the Scottish areas had rates more than twice those in England and Wales. Among the English and Welsh areas, the Salford rate at 44 per 100 000 was highest, followed by Camberwell at 33 and Cardiff at 28 per 100 000. Southampton, Worcester and Oxford had rates lower than the national figure.

TABLE 10

Resident in-patients, 31 December 1983, by length of stay and age – rates per 100 000 total population

| | Length of stay in years, by age group | | | | | | | | | | | |
| | 15–64 | | | | 65 and over | | | | 15 and over | | | |
	<1	1–5	5 and over	Total	<1	1–5	5 and over	Total	<1	1–5	5 and over	Total
Camberwell	71	24	25	120	40	33	47	120	111	57	72	241
Salford	35	22	41	98	29	44	60	133	64	66	102	231
Cardiff	33	13	25	71	30	28	35	92	63	40	59	163
Southampton	29	13	23	65	30	17	18	65	59	30	41	130
Worcester	20	2	17	39	23	13	34	71	43	15	52	110
Oxford	21	5	6	32	17	12	11	40	38	17	18	72
England	29	12	23	65	27	24	31	82	56	36	55	147
Wales	30	12	25	67	28	23	32	82	59	34	57	150
Aberdeen	41	28	35	103	50	64	50	165	91	92	85	268
Scotland	42	26	49	118	48	59	77	184	91	85	126	302

In the very-long-stay group, Salford among English and Welsh registers had the highest rate for patients aged 15–64. At 41 per 100 000 it was 78% higher than the rate for England. Aberdeen also had a high rate although considerably lower than that of Salford. Southampton, Cardiff and Camberwell all had rates similar to that for England, while in Worcester and Oxford rates were lower. In the elderly age group, Salford again had a high rate at 60 per 100 000. Camberwell, Salford, Aberdeen and all Scotland also had high rates compared with England, while Southampton and Oxford had lower rates than England.

Thus the high overall rate in Camberwell was due especially to the short-stay 15–64-year-old subgroup, while in Salford the very-long-stay elderly rate was especially high. In Southampton the elderly long-stay rates were particularly low, while in Worcester the elderly very-long-stay had rates close to the national figure, and most of the other rates, especially for the medium-long-stay, were low. Rates in Oxford were low in all categories but especially the long-stay.

Table 11 shows the percentage breakdown of bed use by age and length of stay at the end of 1983. The elderly occupied at least half the beds in all areas. In Worcester the proportion was almost two-thirds, mainly because of the closure of Powick Hospital (see Chapter 5) to admissions in 1978 and the consequent aging of the residual population, together with low rates for people joining the long-stay population. In Camberwell and Southampton bed use was split evenly between the two age groups. In Southampton this was in part because of policies that try to prevent long-term hospital care for the elderly by the use of community care and relief admissions. Looking at use by length of stay shows that around a third of beds were occupied by the very-long-stay, although this proportion was higher in Worcester and Salford and lower in Oxford. Around a quarter of patients had been in hospital for between one and five years except in Worcester, where the proportion was only one in seven, and Aberdeen where a third of patients were in this category. The majority of long-stay patients were elderly, whereas the short-stay were more equally divided by age.

Table 12 shows the percentage change in rates by length of stay and age group between 31 December 1977 and 31 December 1983. Overall, rates fell by 12–22% except in Camberwell and Salford where the rate rose 7% and Aberdeen where the rate fell only 3%. Falls were largest in the very-long-stay group with a fairly consistent downward trend. In the medium-long-stay group some areas experienced falls in rate while others experienced quite substantial rises.

TABLE 11

Percentage of total occupied beds occupied by patients in each length-of-stay and age group, 31 December 1983

| | Length of stay in years, by age group | | | | | | | | | | | |
| | 15–64 | | | | 65 and over | | | | 15 and over | | | |
	<1	1–5	5 and over	Total	<1	1–5	5 and over	Total	<1	1–5	5 and over	Total
Worcester	18	2	16	36	21	12	31	64	39	14	47	100
Aberdeen	15	10	13	39	19	24	19	61	34	34	32	100
Salford	15	9	18	42	12	19	26	58	28	28	44	100
Cardiff	20	8	15	43	18	17	21	57	39	25	37	100
Oxford	29	6	9	44	23	17	16	56	52	23	25	100
Camberwell	30	10	10	50	17	14	20	50	46	24	30	100
Southampton	22	10	17	50	23	13	14	50	45	23	31	100

TABLE 12
Percentage change[1] in rates 1977–83 by length of stay and age group

		15–64				65 and over				15 and over		
	<1	1–5	5 and over	Total	<1	1–5	5 and over	Total	<1	1–5	5 and over	Total
Camberwell	+ 2	+ 37	− 42	− 7	− 28	+ 3	− 30	− 22	− 11	+ 15	− 34	+ 7
Salford	+ 30	+ 1	− 28	− 7	+ 14	+ 49	+ 5	+ 19	+ 22	+ 34	− 11	+ 7
Southampton	− 28	− 10	− 18	− 22	0	− 5	− 14	− 6	− 16	− 8	− 17	− 14
Cardiff	+ 5	− 16	− 32	− 15	+ 7	− 37	+ 13	− 10	+ 6	− 32	− 12	− 12
Worcester	+ 32	− 80	− 28	− 21	+ 29	− 30	− 37	− 23	+ 31	− 48	− 34	− 22
Oxford	− 30	− 48	− 33	− 34	+ 26	+ 7	− 43	− 10	− 13	− 16	− 40	− 22
Aberdeen	− 6	− 11	− 27	− 15	+ 59	+ 23	− 28	+ 7	+ 21	+ 11	− 28	− 3
Maximum fall	− 30	− 80	− 42	− 34	− 28	− 37	− 43	− 23	− 16	− 48	− 40	− 22
Max. rise/ min. fall	+ 32	+ 37	− 18	− 7	+ 59	+ 49	+ 13	+ 19	+ 31	+ 34	− 11	+ 7

Length of stay in years, by age group

1. Calculated using rates per 100 000 correct to one decimal place.

Usually there were smaller falls or larger rises in the elderly age group than in the younger. All areas except Camberwell and Southampton saw a rise in the elderly short-stay rate over this period, while in the younger age group the pattern was again mixed.

Table 13 shows rates of patients joining the medium-long-stay group (i.e. patients who at 31 December had been in hospital for at least one but less than two years). The area rates come in a similar order to those in Table 10, with Aberdeen the highest, followed by Salford and Camberwell, then Cardiff and Southampton and lastly Worcester and Oxford. Differences between areas were wider, however, with a fivefold difference between the Aberdeen rate of 36 per 100 000 and the rate of 7 per 100 000 in Worcester and Oxford. Rates in the elderly age group were generally higher than in the younger, except in the case of Camberwell and Southampton. There were no marked trends, although a downward trend was rather more common than an upward trend, especially in the younger age group.

Table 14 allows some aspects of the dynamics of the medium-long-stay group at 31 December 1977 and 1982 to be examined. All those aged 15 and over were included. 'Joiners' are those who (as in Table 13) had been in hospital for between one and two years and who therefore joined the medium-long-stay group (between one and five years) during the current year. Table 14 shows that the proportion

TABLE 13
Resident in-patients joining the medium-long-stay group[1], 31 December 1977, 1980 and 1983, by age group – rates per 100 000 total population

	15–64			65 and over			15 and over		
	1977	1980	1983	1977	1980	1983	1977	1980	1983
Aberdeen	12	9	11	18	17	25	29	26	36
Salford	10	8	10	12	16	14	22	24	24
Camberwell	10	12	9	10	12	11	21	24	19
Cardiff	4	6	4	11	15	10	15	21	14
Southampton	8	6	5	8	6	5	16	12	11
Worcester	3	2	1	7	7	6	10	9	7
Oxford	4	2	2	4	6	5	8	8	7

1. Patients resident on 31 December for at least one but less than two years.

TABLE 14

Medium-long-stay (1–5 years) resident in-patients, 31 December 1977 and 1982 – percentages joining, leaving, staying in or graduating from the group

	31 December 1977				31 December 1982			
	Joiners[1]	*Leavers*[2]	*Stayers*[3]	*Graduates*[4]	*Joiners*	*Leavers*	*Stayers*	*Graduates*
Camberwell	41	37	54	9	49	34	63	3
Salford	43	13	77	11	43	23	66	10
Southampton	49	34	55	10	38	27	63	11
Cardiff	25	22	64	13	36	31	58	10
Worcester	34	30	52	20	37	40	43	18
Oxford	42	27	61	12	40	32	56	11

1. Becoming a medium-long-stay patient in 1977 or 1982.
2. Leaving the group through discharge or death during 1978 or 1983.
3. Remaining a medium-long-stay patient until 31 December 1978 or 1983.
4. Remaining in hospital, but 'graduating' to become a very-long-stay patient as of 31 December 1978 or 1983.

of joiners varied from 25% to 50% in 1977 and from 35% to 50% in 1982. In 1977 Cardiff and Worcester had noticeably lower proportions of joiners. There was no clear trend between 1977 and 1982.

The other columns of Table 14 show various outcomes for the medium-long-stay group during the following year (1978 and 1983 respectively). The proportion leaving through discharge or death in the following year ranged from 20% to 40% except in Salford in 1978. There was a tendency for the proportion leaving to rise slightly between 1978 and 1983. Typically, in 1983 just over 70% of the discharges and deaths from the 1–5-year group were elderly, although the proportion in Camberwell was slightly lower, at 64%. At least half the patients were still in the 1–5-year group at the end of 1978, although in Salford the proportion was 77%. Around 60% of the 1982 group 'stayed' to the end of 1983, except in Worcester where the figure was 43%. In both years, in most areas, just over 10% 'graduated' to the very-long-stay group; the exceptions were Worcester (around 20%) and Camberwell (3% in 1983).

Table 15 shows rates for patients joining the very-long-stay group. That is, at 31 December they had been in hospital for at least five but less than six years. Rates were not of the same order as in Tables 10 and 13, since in 1983 Camberwell had a low rate and in Worcester the rate was above both Camberwell and Southampton. Rates per 100 000 total population ranged from 11 down to less than one. Aberdeen and Salford and, in some categories, Cardiff had the highest

TABLE 15

Resident in-patients joining the very-long-stay group (patients resident in hospital on 31 December for at least five but less than six years) – rates per 100 000 total population, by age group and year

	15–64			65 and over			15 and over		
	1977	*1980*	*1983*	*1977*	*1980*	*1983*	*1977*	*1980*	*1983*
Aberdeen	3	2	4	6	7	5	9	9	9
Salford	3	3	1	3	6	5	6	8	6
Cardiff	2	2	1	3	9	3	5	11	4
Worcester	1	−[1]	1	4	2	2	5	2	4
Southampton	1	2	1	1	1	2	3	3	3
Camberwell	2	1	1	4	4	1	7	5	2
Oxford	−[1]	−[1]	1	1	1	1	1	1	2

1. Rate < 0.5.

TABLE 16

Percentage of very-long-stay resident in-patients joining in year to 31 December 1977 and 1982, and leaving through death or discharge during following year

	% joining in 1977	% leaving in 1978				% joining in 1982	% leaving in 1983		
	15 and over	15 and over	15–64	65 and over		15 and over	15 and over	15–64	65 and over
Camberwell	6	12	12	12		5	10	6	12
Salford	5	10	7	13		8	16	7	19
Southampton	6	14	7	23		2	11	2	22
Cardiff	8	10	5	15		10	13	1	21
Worcester	6	11	8	12		5	10	5	13
Oxford	4	12	4	16		7	11	3	15

TABLE 17

Very-long-stay (> 5 years) resident in-patients on 31 December 1983, aged over 65 – total numbers and percentage aged under 65 at start of current in-patient stay, by clinical group[1]

	Percentage admitted before age 65					Numbers (%)				
	SP	AF	DM	OT	Total	SP	AF	DM	OT	Total
Camberwell	97	80	38	80	86	39(68)	5(9)	8(14)	5(9)	57(100)
Salford	94	43	21	68	72	77(53)	23(16)	19(13)	25(17)	144(100)
Southampton	94	100	50	62	78	17(47)	4(11)	2(6)	13(36)	36(100)
Cardiff	87	89	11	23	64	54(57)	9(10)	18(19)	13(14)	94(100)
Worcester	99	83	14	81	84	72(63)	12(11)	14(12)	16(14)	114(100)
Oxford	90	63	13	92	76	29(50)	8(14)	8(14)	13(22)	58(100)
Aberdeen	98	59	16	80	70	112(41)	46(17)	58(21)	55(20)	271(100)

1. See footnote to Table 5.

rates. Rates were higher and more variable in the elderly age group. In 1983 the rate for the younger age group was 1 per 100 000 in all areas except Aberdeen.

Table 16 shows the percentage (as of 31 December) of the long-stay group who joined in 1977 and 1982, and the percentage who left through discharge or death during 1978 and 1983, respectively. The 'leavers' are tabulated by age and the percentages calculated on the number of resident in-patients in each age group. Around 4–8% of the very-long-stay group joined during the current year, although in 1982 the Southampton figure was much lower at 2% and the Cardiff figure rather higher at 10%. There was no clear difference in the percentage joining in the two years. From 10% to 16% of the very-long-stay group left each year through discharge or death, and again there was little difference between the two years. There were, however, considerable differences between the age groups. Less than 8% of the younger age group left through discharge or death during the year (except in 1978 in Camberwell), compared with 12–23% of the elderly.

It is difficult to distinguish between those elderly in-patients who are suffering from the diseases of old age (whose numbers are likely to be related to the population of elderly people in the community and the provision of psychogeriatric services) and those who have become old in hospital, having been admitted many years before, with other functional or organic illnesses not specific to old age. The numbers in this latter group will tend to decline as patients die or are discharged. Table 17 is an attempt to distinguish these two groups by calculating the percentage of very-long-stay elderly patients who were aged under 65 at the start of their current admission.

Table 17 shows that at least two-thirds of the elderly very-long-stay patients were admitted before their 65th birthday and that this proportion rises to 85% in Camberwell and Worcester. Except in Cardiff, 90% or more of the elderly very-long-stay schizophrenic patients were admitted before age 65. Similarly, with only two exceptions, the majority in the depressive ('AF') and other ('OT') categories were admitted before age 65. As one would expect, most patients with dementia ('DM') were admitted after 65, although in Southampton and Camberwell the proportion was lower than elsewhere. Table 17 also shows the numbers and percentage distribution of the elderly very-long-stay patients by clinical group. There are interesting differences in the percentage of this group who are demented. In most areas the proportion is around 12–14%, but in Cardiff and Aberdeen the proportion is around 20% while in Southampton the very low proportion of 6% is probably explained by the local policy of trying to keep demented patients out of long-stay care until a late stage in their illness (see also Chapter 7).

Table 18 shows, for all long-stay (over one year) in-patients, some more detailed information on age and clinical group. Leaving aside Southampton, which does not fit the pattern of the other areas, the 15–64 age group comprised 32–47% of the total long-stay population in 1977. In all areas except Camberwell this proportion fell after 1977, so that by 1983 the range was 30–38%. No more than a third and usually less than a quarter of the 15–64 age group were

TABLE 18

Long-stay (> 1 year) resident in-patients (aged 15 and over), 31 December 1977 and 1983 – rates per 100 000 total population, and percentage distribution by age group

| | Rates | | Percentage by age group | | | | | | | |
| | | | 15–44 | | 45–64 | | 65–74 | | 75 and over | |
	1977	1983	1977	1983	1977	1983	1977	1983	1977	1983
Camberwell	160	129	11	13	26	25	25	20	38	42
Salford	165	168	7	7	40	31	27	23	26	39
Southampton	81	71	11	15	42	36	18	22	30	27
Cardiff	126	100	11	7	30	30	24	24	35	39
Worcester	108	67	5	2	27	28	31	24	37	46
Oxford	50	35	8	8	30	24	27	21	36	47
Aberdeen	201	177	11	8	28	27	24	18	36	47

TABLE 19

Numbers of long-stay resident in-patients (aged 15 and over) and percentage distribution by clinical group, 31 December 1977 and 1983

| | Numbers | | Percentage distribution by clinical group[1] | | | | | | | |
| | | | SP | | AF | | DM | | OT[2] | |
	1977	1983	1977	1983	1977	1983	1977	1983	1977	1983
Camberwell	218	156	60	59	10	10	19	15	11	11
Salford	426	397	55	47	12	13	12	18	22	30
Southampton	170	144	47	47	16	10	16	19	17	25
Cardiff	353	270	48	47	5	9	31	29	16	15
Worcester	343	224	52	52	8	8	20	26	19	14
Oxford	245	177	43	38	11	10	22	31	24	22
Aberdeen	1018	952	38	32	15	14	24	34	23	16

1. See footnote to Table 5.
2. Here includes alcohol- and drug-related disorders.

aged under 45. There were no clear trends in the percentage aged 15–44, but the proportion aged 45–64 fell or was constant between 1977 and 1983 in almost all areas. As the proportion aged 15–64 fell, so the proportion who were aged over 65 rose, but this increase, except in Southampton, was concentrated entirely in the over 75 age group which, by 1983 made up 40% or more of all long-stay patients. The proportion aged 65–74 fell. In Southampton the pattern was different, with the proportions aged 15–64 and 65–74 rising, while the proportions aged 45–64 and 75 and over fell. Southampton also had a higher proportion aged 15–64 than other areas (15%) and a lower proportion aged 75 and over.

Table 19 shows the percentage distribution of all long-stay patients by clinical group. In most areas about half the long-stay patients had diagnoses of schizophrenia or paranoid states ('SP'), about 10% had an affective disorder ('AF'), and around 20% had dementia ('DM'). In Oxford and Aberdeen, the proportion of schizophrenia was lower and the proportion of dementia higher. Between 1977 and 1983, three areas saw substantial falls in the proportion of schizophrenia and in no area did the proportion rise. In five of the seven areas the proportion of dementia rose, often by substantial amounts.

All the tables so far have employed the 'continuous-stay' definition of length of stay. It can be argued, however, that it is clinically more meaningful to ignore short breaks in care, for example when a patient is placed unsuccessfully in a hostel for a brief time or goes to a general hospital for an operation. To adopt a strict continuous-stay definition means that a patient who had been in hospital many years would be classified as a short-stay patient in the period after such a readmission. In Table 20, the length-of-stay distributions have ignored any breaks in in-patient care of less than 30 days. This means that if a patient was admitted, stayed five years, and then left the hospital but was readmitted within 30 days, it would be the first admission five years earlier, not the recent readmission, that would serve as the starting point for calculating length of stay. This method will result in fewer short-stay patients and more very-long-stay patients compared with the 'continuous-stay' method. The effect on medium-long-stay numbers could be either positive or negative. In order to calculate the effect on length of stay of ignoring breaks in care, a full in-patient history is needed for at least five years. This condition was met by 1980 in Camberwell, Oxford and Southampton,

TABLE 20

Percentage change (compared with 'continuous' method) in number of resident in-patients aged 15 and over in each length-of-stay group when breaks in care of less than 30 days are ignored

	< 1 year				1–5 years				5 years and over			
	1980	1981	1982	1983	1980	1981	1982	1983	1980	1981	1982	1983
Camberwell	−7	−8	−4	−4	−2	0	−14	−14	+11	+11	+11	+18
Oxford	−2	−4	−6	−5	−5	−9	+2	+6	+9	+10	+5	+2
Southampton	−3	−1	−4	−5	−1	0	+7	+4	+3	+7	+6	+7
Salford	−	0	−3	−3	0	−1	+1	+1	−	*	+1	+1
Cardiff	−	−	−	−9	−	−	−	+6	−	−	−	+6

−, data not available.
*, less than 0.5%.

by 1981 in Salford (because of the 1975 expansion of the register), and by 1983 in Cardiff (since accurate admission data were only available from 1978). It is theoretically possible that ignoring short breaks in care can result in a series of short admissions being linked together so as to appear to constitute one long in-patient stay, but this is likely to happen only rarely when the break ignored is 30 days or less.

Table 20 shows the percentage difference between the numbers in each length-of-stay group, calculated by ignoring breaks of less than 30 days, and the numbers found by the continuous-stay method of calculation. The largest differences occurred in Camberwell, where ignoring breaks in care led to increases of up to 18% in the very-long-stay category. In all the other areas differences were 10% or less and very small differences of under 3% were common, especially in Salford.

Summary

Admission rates in most areas were higher than for England as a whole. Admission rates for the younger age group had, generally, declined between 1977 and 1983, while in the elderly age group most areas had experienced a substantial rise. The admission rate of the elderly was about twice that of the younger age group and they stayed in hospital longer. Variations in the number of admissions per person admitted cannot explain the variation in admission rates. There was a threefold variation between register areas in admission rates for schizophrenia and for dementia.

Resident in-patient rates in English and Welsh areas were largely correlated with the social and demographic character of the areas, with exceptions in particular age or length-of-stay groups being explicable in terms of local circumstance or policy. At least half the beds were occupied by the elderly, this figure rising in some areas to two-thirds. Well over half the beds were occupied by long-stay patients, to a maximum of 70%. The majority of long stay patients were elderly while the short-stay patients were more equally divided by age. Overall, resident in-patient rates fell by 10–20% from 1977 to 1983. Falls were generally larger and more consistently downward in the very-long-stay group than in other groups where no clear trends were discernible, apart from elderly short-stay rates, which rose in most areas.

There were very wide differences in rates of 'recruitment' to the medium-long-stay (1–5 year) group, though the areas were in the same order as for the overall resident in-patient rates. At least a third and up to half of the medium-long-stay group joined the group each year, between 20% and 40% left through discharge or death, and about 10% went on to the very-long-stay group. From 4% to 8% of the very-long-stay group joined each year and 10–15% left through discharge or death, although this proportion was higher among the elderly.

At least two-thirds and up to 85% of all the elderly very-long-stay and over 90% of elderly people with schizophrenia were last admitted before their 65th birthday. The rise in the proportion of elderly long-stay patients was confined to those aged 75 and over and was probably related to increases in the proportion of dementia. A change in the definition of length of stay such that short breaks in care were ignored made little difference to the numbers in each length-of-stay group, except in Camberwell.

Reference

GIBBONS, J., JENNINGS, C. & WING, J. K. (1984) *Psychiatric Care in Eight Register Areas.* Southampton: University Department of Psychiatry. (Copies obtainable by sending £2.50, cheque payable to University of Southampton, to University Department of Psychiatry, Royal South Hants Hospital, Southampton SO9 4PE.)

3 A decade of mental health care in an English urban community: patterns and trends in Salford, 1976–87

TOM FRYERS and KATE WOOFF

The psychiatric case register

The first psychiatric case register in Salford started in 1959, linked to the development programme for the Atlas computer (Adelstein *et al*, 1968; Susser, 1968; Susser *et al*, 1969, 1970). Its pioneering work was cut short in 1964 by loss of staff and funding. The present register commenced with a census of all Salford people currently receiving psychiatric or other 'mental health' care on 1 January 1968 (Fryers *et al*, 1970). It was intended both as a service information system, and a research facility (Fryers, 1976a, b, 1979a, 1986a). To this end, its data set, codes, classifications and processes were largely modelled upon the Camberwell case register, which had started in 1964 (Wing & Hailey, 1972). The potential for comparative studies was demonstrated by the first ten-year analyses (Wing & Fryers, 1976).

Salford Metropolitan District is a largely urban segment of the Greater Manchester conurbation in the north-west of England. With a population of about a quarter of a million, it was formed in 1974 from two adjacent areas. Salford County Borough (Salford East), an administrative entity for health and welfare for over 100 years, was 'inner-city' urban, and environmentally impoverished, with a population of generally low socio-economic status, reducing from almost 250 000 in 1931 to under 100 000 in 1981. The added area (Salford West) was largely suburban, environmentally and socially more balanced, with a population rapidly increasing until recent years. The contrasting demographic histories and characters of the two 'halves' of Salford are matched by different mental health service traditions, thus presenting unusual opportunities for comparison within the register population base.

The context in which the register started and flourished was almost unique in Britain. An extensive community-based service had been built up since the late 1950s, which included a variety of day and residential care, and was founded upon a large body of trained and experienced specialist mental health social workers, who supported people at home and elsewhere, handled most emergencies, and liaised with psychiatrists and other hospital-based professional staff. The degree of co-operation between the local authority mental health department and hospital psychiatric service staff was such that it was not unrealistic to speak of a single or unified Salford service. However, many aspects of the service remained inadequate, and one of the purposes of the register was to monitor progressive developments of the community-based service (Susser, 1968; Mountney *et al*, 1969; Freeman, 1979; Wooff *et al*, 1983).

Since its inception, the Salford register has continuously collected comprehensive data in spite of several administrative upheavals affecting the mental health services. National reorganisation of personal social services in 1971 led to the creation of a single generic social work agency in the local authority, and made 'mental health care' difficult to define and identify. In 1974 the population base of 138 000 in the county borough was increased to 270 000 with the creation of the new Salford Metropolitan District (Salford MD – Salford East and West). At the same time, the National Health Service was thoroughly reorganised, again changing the service context in which the register operated, and the relationship to both management and clinical personnel.

The Salford register has several peculiar characteristics. It has now collected data on virtually all mental health service contacts of the Salford East population for 20 years, and of the Salford West population for 13 years. Since these two populations have very different demographic and service histories, they offer considerable potential for 'internal' comparison. The administrative upheavals that have made life difficult have also provided almost 'experimental' changes to monitor. Throughout these changes, it has recorded not only episodes of care given by specialist mental health social workers, but also 'mental health' care given by generic social workers. It has also been possible to monitor the effects of major developments, such as the establishment of a community psychiatric nursing service and a specialist psychogeriatric service. Services for Salford are geographically compact and administratively cohesive, and there is almost no private care of any type, so that the register can claim virtually comprehensive coverage of all mental health care outside primary medical services. Although the register serves a multiagency, multiprofessional service complex, access to personal information is carefully controlled, and in its long history, we have never faced any serious issue of confidentiality or privacy.

Basic measures of service use

The data presented are intended to illustrate both the uses of a register and the patterns of service use revealed by the register in Salford. Data on types of care routinely collected are: admission to and discharge from in-patient care and other specified residential care; specialist National Health Service and local authority day care; mental health social work care; and community psychiatric nursing care. All out-patients and other face-to-face contacts with psychiatrists at any site are recorded, as well as all nursing contacts for injection of depot neuroleptics. All such services providing for any resident of Salford, inside or outside the city boundaries, are included, excepting only occasional patients attending some rarely used facilities in other districts. Diagnoses (up to three recorded at any one time) are those assigned by the psychiatrists. They are coded and stored individually, but are usually analysed in 11 main categories (Wing, 1970).

Point prevalence is the simplest statistic used. This represents a census or cross-sectional analysis of people in receipt of any of the above services on 1 January each year. Those in residential care are easily defined; those in day care are currently experiencing a 'spell' of day care, not necessarily attending every day;

a similar definition applies to social work care; for out-patient and similar consultations, and domiciliary visits by doctors or nurses, an artificial definition is imposed on the contact data requiring contacts before and after the census point, with no more than 91 days ('three months') between them.

Point-prevalence data are limited in their ability adequately to describe a service situation when duration of episode is as variable as in mental health care. In this field therefore, period prevalence (usually year prevalence) proves instructive. For this, persons identified on the census at the beginning of each year are added to all other persons who make contact with any service during the ensuing year. This hybrid statistic thus represents all people contacting the services in any period of 12 months.

In describing the simple outlines of a population service it is necessary to use incidence statistics, which pose some difficulties. The real onset of psychiatric disorder is often difficult to establish, may long antedate any seeking for help, and may be unrecognised, unrecorded or inaccessible in primary medical or generic social work services. New cases to the specialist services, and therefore to the register, are the easiest to handle, but history of previous contact, before the register started, or in another community, is not easy to obtain consistently and reliably. However, only the first few years of a register are unreliable with regard to inceptors, and we believe that all new registrations with no positive previous history recorded represent a reasonable approximation to true inceptions of serious mental illness in Salford.

The statistics can reveal the patterns of any one form of care, such as in-patient care, any group of facilities, such as day care, any type of personnel, such as social workers, or of all facilities together. A service which offered little more than admission to a large mental hospital would be very easy to record and monitor, but as a community service becomes more diverse, more dispersed, more multidisciplinary, less formal, and less segregated, recording and monitoring become progressively more difficult and more dependent upon modern information technology. Thus the provision of information, monitoring, audit, evaluation and research become more demanding of time, money and specialist skills.

The analysis of trends over many years, and comparisons between groups defined by age, sex, diagnosis, domicile and other variables renders much valuable information, even with the simple measures outlined above, but many other statistics and methods of analysis are available. Among the most valuable are cohort studies, since registers are peculiarly able to follow up defined groups of people across contacts with many agencies, facilities and personnel, and over many years. Of course, studies requiring additional data to those routinely collected may readily be mounted upon the register's existing system.

Point prevalence: censuses in Salford Metropolitan District 1976–87

Figure 2 shows the trends in the age-specific population rate (per 1000) for all services and all Salford, in three broad age groups. The range of services includes mental health contacts with community nurses and social workers, 'injection only' visits, and day centres, as well as out-patient and in-patient hospital and

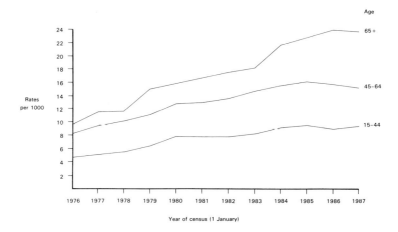

Fig. 2. Point prevalence (all Salford services) 1976–87. Age-specific rates per 1000 population, Salford MD

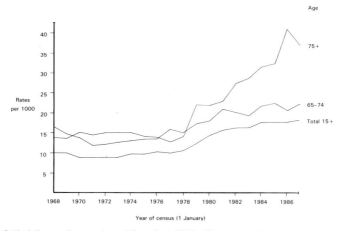

Fig. 3. Salford East, point prevalence (all services) 1968–87. Age-specific rates per 1000 population

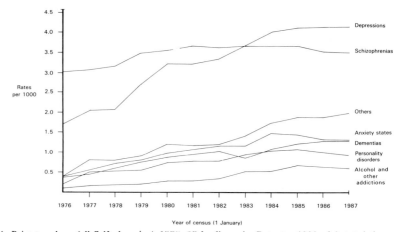

Fig. 4. Point prevalence (all Salford services) 1976–87 by diagnosis. Rates per 1000 adult population

psychiatrist contacts; psychologist contacts were not included. Throughout the period, higher prevalence has been associated with greater age, but the outstanding feature is that all at least doubled in ten years, those over 65 years old having more than doubled. The figures for the last few years suggest a plateau at all ages, but it will be some years before this pattern could be confirmed.

Figure 3 shows that, at least for Salford East, where we have continuous data since 1968, the increase in prevalence has only been experienced since 1978. In the ten years before that, there was remarkably little change in any age group. Figure 3 shows separate age-specific prevalence rates for those aged 65–74, and for those aged 75 years or over. It is clear that, although the increase applies to all age groups, it is most prominent in the oldest. In 1987, almost 2.5% of the population aged 65 years or over, and 4% of those aged 75 years or over, were receiving formal mental health care at any one time.

Figure 4 shows the trends in certain diagnostic groups expressed as rates in the adult (15 years and over) population. All have increased, but not equally. Schizophrenia has changed least. After a modest rise of about 20% in the first five years from 1976, it has been remarkably stable at about 3.6 per 1000 adult population. The earlier rise may well reflect the time taken to accumulate new cases of a chronic and recurrent disorder like schizophrenia after the expansion of the register's coverage to Salford West in 1975. Depressions, on the other hand, have increased consistently over 11 years, to approximately 150% of the prevalence in 1976. Dementias, almost wholly in old age, have increased by over 200%. These rates take account of the changes in population age structure: the increase in the *numbers* of people with dementia at the beginning of each year was even greater. However, it should be noted that the figures for dementia remain very much smaller than those for depressions.

The diagnostic groups 'anxiety states' and 'personality disorders' also increased substantially from 1976, but have appeared to level off in recent years. The greatest proportional increases were seen in disorders related to alcohol and other drugs, but from very small beginnings in 1976. The balance of disorders within the total census population has changed. In 1976 schizophrenia accounted for 44% of all those receiving care at one time, but this has reduced to 25%. Depressions include relatively few severe disorders, but many mild and unspecified disorders, and feature particularly prominently in out-patient figures. Grouped together, they increased from 25% to 30% of the whole census count. Although dementias increased greatly, they still constituted only 9% in 1987.

The fact that the substantial increases in prevalence occurred throughout the 11-year period in virtually all diagnostic groups, including the group 'other' (which constituted many small groups) suggests that *general* factors may be the most important determinants, rather than any specific factors related to specific types of disorder. Because of the nature of census definitions, such increases in *point prevalence* can result from more people in contact, longer periods of contact, or more contacts per person, each leading to more people fulfilling the 91-day criterion for the census. The increases probably reflect the expanding and diversifying mental health care system, and a general trend towards seeking, or accepting, formal mental health care more readily, and for a wider spectrum of symptoms. It could also reflect increased stresses in urban society in the last ten years, related to unemployment, poor housing, relative poverty, and a generally impoverished environment, but this is difficult to demonstrate.

TABLE 21

Salford MD: Point prevalence on 1 January for all services, 1976–87 – numbers, and age- and sex-specific rates per 1000 adult (15 +) population

		1976		1979		1983		1987	
Age		*No.*	*Rate*	*No.*	*Rate*	*No.*	*Rate*	*No.*	*Rate*
15–44	Male	232	4.48	324	6.42	378	7.08	443	8.49
	Female	251	5.04	321	6.65	480	9.58	514	10.45
45–64	Male	246	7.93	296	10.16	351	12.72	315	12.30
	Female	301	9.19	386	12.70	474	16.63	471	17.98
65 and over	Male	107	7.85	164	11.63	191	13.45	254	17.16
	Female	255	10.96	403	16.99	511	21.29	669	27.31
Total (rates	Male	585	6.06	784	8.32	920	9.66	1013	10.94
per 1000 adults)	Female	807	7.63	1110	10.75	1465	14.28	1655	16.57
Total (rates	Male		4.60		6.44		7.71		8.83
per 1000 all ages)	Female		5.99		8.58		11.66		13.64

The increases certainly do reflect an increased work load on the service as a whole, and an extension of the range and diversity of facilities and personnel available.

Table 21 reveals interesting differences in the sexes at different ages by comparing censuses from 1976, 1979, 1983, and 1987. There were higher numbers and rates for women at all ages, the difference increasing with age. The latest disparity in numbers is especially striking; women dominate the psychogeriatric service. The changing distribution of three important diagnoses by sex is shown in Table 22. In schizophrenia men and women have shown very similar rates throughout the 11 years, but in depressions and dementias, population rates for women have been consistently between two and three times those for men. The excess of women in the totals has increased considerably; by 1987 it was over 50%.

TABLE 22

Salford MD: Point prevalence on 1 January for all services, 1976–87 – numbers and rates per 1000 adult population: sex and diagnosis

	1976		1979		1983		1987	
Diagnosis	*No.*	*Rate*	*No.*	*Rate*	*No.*	*Rate*	*No.*	*Rate*
Schizophrenias								
Male	311	3.22	345	3.66	347	3.64	343	3.70
Female	340	2.87	345	3.34	358	3.49	332	3.32
Depressions								
Male	98	1.02	165	1.75	195	2.05	201	2.17
Female	252	2.38	375	3.63	514	5.01	594	5.95
Dementias								
Male	20	0.21	49	0.52	48	0.50	60	0.65
Female	59	0.56	113	1.09	137	1.34	186	1.86
Others								
Male	156	1.62	225	2.39	330	3.47	409	4.42
Female	192	1.81	277	2.68	456	4.44	543	5.44
Total								
Male	585	6.06	784	8.32	920	9.66	1013	10.94
Female	807	7.63	1110	10.75	1465	14.28	1655	16.53

Year prevalence, 1976–86: the total burden of illness

Year prevalence statistics show the total number of individuals who have had any sort of contact with the services within one year. They therefore reflect more satisfactorily the total burden of illness in the community and the total burden of care on the services. Figure 5 gives details of the age distribution and shows several important features. All age groups between 35 and 74 have shown rather similar age-specific rates, which have been slowly and steadily rising. In general, the increase in this broad age band was from a range of 17–22 per 1000 in 1976, to 26–32 per 1000 in 1986. The 25–34 age group was at the top of this range in 1976 at about 22 per 1000, but increased very little, to about 24 per 1000 in 1986. In contrast, the 15–24 age group remained at about 11–12 per 1000 throughout.

At the other end of the age scale, those aged 75 and over increased in number dramatically from 19 per 1000 in 1976 to over 66 per 1000 in 1986. The greatest increase was from 1981, following the appointment of a new specialist psychogeriatrician. The figures illustrate the value of monitoring new developments, but the earlier increase in this age group shows the reasons for establishing the new service, and the numbers in this group have continued to increase annually, although less dramatically recently. These high rates represent a major component of mental health care; the 1057 individuals aged 75 and over in 1986 constituted almost 20% of all people making contact during that year.

The increases in year prevalence also reflect other increases in service provision. There was little community psychiatric nursing in 1976, but throughout the 1980s this has contributed a substantial and increasing component to the year-prevalence figures (Wooff *et al*, 1986). Over the same period of time, contacts with all services monitored by the register increased. In general, our experience has been that additions and extensions to the range of treatment, care and support that are provided, add both to the numbers of people receiving help and the average length of periods of help. In one sense this must necessarily reflect unmet need, but it may also reflect inappropriate services, inadequate assessment of need and priorities, and lack of a sufficient overview for planning, monitoring

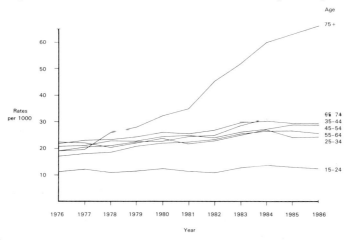

Fig. 5. Year prevalence (all Salford services) 1976–86. Age-specific rates per 1000 population

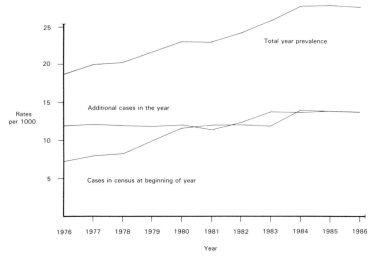

Fig. 6. Year prevalence (all Salford services) 1976–86, by diagnosis. Rates per 1000 adult population

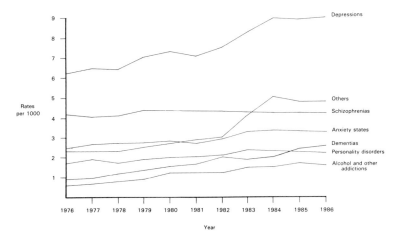

Fig. 7. Components of year prevalence, Salford, 1976–86

and evaluating the community-based service as a whole. As this becomes more and more difficult with increasing diversity of care, the need for new management structures also becomes apparent.

The diagnostic distributions of year prevalence are given in Fig. 6. They are most remarkable for the consistency of the pattern for each group of disorders. There has been virtually no change for schizophrenia, and the increase in 'personality disorder' was slight. Depressions continued to rise substantially, but, not unexpectedly, dementias and alcohol and addictive disorders increased proportionately most. They each more than doubled between 1976 and 1986, but remain small in the total.

Figure 7 clarifies the changing contribution of the two components of year prevalence: persons counted on each annual census, and persons added in the following year. Although in recent years both components have increased slightly together, the increase was entirely due to increases in point prevalence up to 1982. This measure tends to reflect chronic illness, long-term disability, and continuity of care. This reinforces the points made earlier about extensions in the range of care and increased frequency of contact for people with long-term mental disorders. To explore this further we need to look at the rate of inception, that is, the number of people each year presenting to the mental health services for the very first time.

Inceptions, 1976–86: the flow of new cases

Figure 8 gives the annual age-specific rates from 1976 to 1986 for new cases with no known previous history of contact with any mental health service, that is, inception rates. The trends vary with age. In the age groups 15–44 and 45–64 years, inception rates decreased slowly from 1976 to 1982, since when they rose somewhat irregularly, by 1986 back to levels similar to those in 1976. The overall change was very small. The 65–74 age group rose slowly until the new psychogeriatric service boosted inceptions in 1982 and 1983, then remained around the new level of about 7 per 1000 per annum. The over 75 age group exhibited a similar pattern but on a much bigger scale; the rise from 1976 was substantial, that in 1982–83 was dramatic, and the level inceptions apparently settled at was about 20 per 1000 per annum. The 65–74 age group doubled in ten years; the over 75 age group quadrupled in ten years.

The increase in mental health care in Salford, as measured by service-use statistics, has encompassed many more elderly people presenting for the first time, while accepting similar numbers of younger ones, and providing more continuous care to long-established patients. All these figures are population rates, and thus take account of basic demographic changes.

Table 23 shows the inception rates for the two parts of the city with very different population histories, environments and service traditions, as means for two five-year periods up to 1985. Salford East, the 'inner city', has consistently

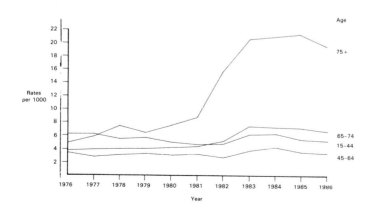

Fig. 8. Annual inceptions (all Salford services), 1976–86. Age-specific rates per 1000 population

TABLE 23

Mean annual inceptions, Salford East and West – age-specific and sex-specific rates per 1000 total and adult population, 1976–80 and 1981–85

	1976–80		1981–85	
	East	West	East	West
Age				
15–44	6.8	5.2	6.7	5.2
45–64	4.6	3.2	4.1	3.5
65 and over	5.3	4.9	11.9	11.6
Rates per 1000 total population				
Male	3.0	3.0	4.6	3.6
Female	4.1	4.2	6.7	5.6
Totals	3.5	3.6	5.7	4.7
Rates per 1000 adult (over 15) population				
Male	4.7	3.8	5.7	4.5
Female	6.5	5.3	8.3	7.0
Totals	5.6	4.6	7.1	5.8

TABLE 24

Mean annual inceptions for Salford East and West, 1976–85 – population rates by diagnostic group

Diagnosis	Rates per 1000 total population		Rates per 1000 adult population	
	East	West	East	West
Depression	1.10	1.11	1.60	1.40
Anxiety state	0.59	0.59	0.79	0.74
Dementia	0.46	0.41	0.64	0.52
Personality disorder	0.39	0.26	0.55	0.33
Alcohol and addictive disorders	0.27	0.17	0.37	0.22
Severe depression	0.10	0.12	0.14	0.15
Schizophrenia	0.11	0.09	0.15	0.11

had higher inception rates for both sexes and all age groups. The table shows that using rates related to total populations may mask real differences because of differences in the proportion of children in each community. In the totals related to the adult population, the difference has been about 20% higher in Salford East, similar for both sexes, although female inceptions in both communities were considerably higher than male inceptions. The difference between East and West varies with age, being greatest in the 15–44 age group, moderate in the 45–64 age group, and very small in the over 65 age group.

Table 24 shows the main diagnostic inception rates as means for the ten-year period 1976–85 for the two communities. Salford East shows higher mean rates for all but severe depression, although the difference is quite small for the largest groups, mild and moderate depression, and anxiety states, and is not large for dementias. The difference is much greater for disorders related to alcohol and drugs, and for personality disorders, which have been increasing fairly dramatically in the East, but much more slowly in the West.

Figure 9 illustrates the similar rates in both communities for the period 1976–86 for depressions and 'other neuroses'. Inceptions of schizophrenia are consistently 50–100% higher in Salford East (the 'inner city') than Salford West, although numbers are, of course, very small. These inception data confirm the differences exhibited by the point-prevalence data.

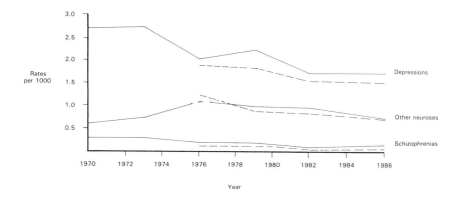

Fig. 9. Salford East (——) and Salford West (- - - -), annual inceptions 1970–86, by diagnosis. Rates per 1000 total population

These two observations from Tables 23 and 24 (the Salford East excess of inceptions in younger adults, and in diagnostic groups 'addictions' and 'personality disorders') may well be related of course, as these diagnoses tend to be more common at these ages, but this does not easily explain the excess being in young women. Salford East is the inner city, subjected over several decades to massive demolition and rehousing, with great disruption of the communities. The differences in inception rates between the two parts of Salford probably reflect differences in social problems and needs: the higher inception rates from Salford East include more new patients who were single, more living alone, and more unemployed than in the West. The data also imply that solutions do not lie entirely within the mental health services, but in wider realms of social policy.

Admissions to hospital: in-patient care

We have seen extensions of 'community' services affecting the population statistics in various ways, but have these developments had any effect on admissions to hospital and length of in-patient stay? The principal provider of hospital care throughout the period studied was the general hospital psychiatric unit, but a very large mental hospital is still used, particularly for longer periods of care. Table 25 gives total admissions and total persons admitted annually from 1976 to 1986 for all Salford. There was some variation in both admissions and persons admitted, but little overall change in the rates per 1000 population until the latter few years, when both tended to increase. With the concurrent fall in population, the rates show a greater recent increase. The lowest figures (for 1979) were associated with local industrial action in that year! Admission rates have been consistently higher from Salford East than Salford West, and in both communities are higher for women (Fryers, 1988a).

Table 26 differentiates between admissions of people aged under and over 65 years. The increase in admissions has actually been limited to those over 65.

TABLE 25

Salford MD: admissions to all psychiatric beds, 1976–86 – numbers and rates per 1000 total population

Year	Admissions		Persons admitted	
	Numbers	Rates	Numbers	Rates
1976	998	3.81	791	3.02
1977	963	3.73	757	2.93
1978	936	3.68	745	2.93
1979	859	3.42	687	2.74
1980	975	3.94	761	3.08
1981	989	4.06	765	3.14
1982	900	3.68	709	2.90
1983	1054	4.30	804	3.28
1984	1103	4.55	826	3.41
1985	1102	4.59	815	3.39
1986	1204	5.05	811	3.40

TABLE 26

Salford MD: admissions to all psychiatric beds, 1977–85 – numbers and age-specific rates per 1000

Year	Numbers		Rates	
	15–64	65 and over	15–64	65 and over
1977	746	217	4.56	5.83
1979	639	218	4.00	5.76
1981	690	299	4.43	7.78
1983	706	348	4.42	9.11
1985	722	380	4.62	9.87

In 1985 this represented approximately 1% of the population over 65. Of course, this increase is related to the excess of women admitted, and the increase in dementia and depressions.

The register records a continuous period of in-patient care even after local transfers between hospitals. Table 27 shows that most patients stay less than one month, and the proportion has varied only between 57% and 65%. There has been little change in those staying between one and three months, varying from 16% to 22%, and not much more in the proportion staying between three months and one year, with a variation of 10–18%, including two extreme years without which the variation is only 12–16%. Few admissions lead to a stay of over a year, varying between 4% and 9%, with an average of 6.25%. The proportion staying at least a year increases with age, and in those aged over 65 years is higher for women, especially in Salford West. In recent years there has been a considerable effort put into rehabilitation, including the establishment of small 'group homes' scattered throughout the community, and many of these have been successful in providing long-term accommodation, with support, for those with no adequate home or family. But in numeric terms they have as yet had little impact on the in-patient service as a whole.

There is a special problem of interpreting data on long-stay in-patients (see Chapter 4). In any community whose population has fallen as dramatically and extensively as Salford East, there will tend to be high point-prevalence rates for any relatively less mobile group. The extreme example is those resident in long-stay institutions. Salford East has, therefore, very high rates for long-stay

TABLE 27
Salford MD: length of stay after admission to any psychiatric bed, 1976–86

Year	Length of stay			
	0–30 days (%)	31–60 days (%)	61–364 days (%)	1 year or more (%)
1976	64	18	10	7
1977	64	17	13	6
1978	63	17	13	6
1979	60	19	12	9
1980	63	18	12	6
1981	62	16	15	8
1982	58	18	18	7
1983	62	16	15	6
1984	62	16	15	6
1985	57	22	16	5
1986	61	19	15	5
1987	65	17	14	4

in-patients, but Salford West has low rates because it has had an increasing population. The difference applies to both sexes and all ages, but decreases with age. Similar phenomena are found elsewhere: Camberwell has high rates, Oxford has low rates (Gibbons *et al*, 1984).

Numbers and rates for lengths of stay over ten years have been diminishing, mostly by death. For lengths of stay of one to ten years, representing relatively recent accumulation of 'new long-stay' patients, there are striking differences between age groups. Rates for men aged 15–44 have been steadily falling; those

TABLE 28
Salford East and Salford West: admissions to all psychiatric beds, 1968–82 – rates per 1000 adult population, by diagnosis

Diagnosis	1968	1974	1979	1982	1986
Schizophrenias					
Salford East	1.38	1.09	1.01	1.04	0.96
Salford West	–	–	0.51	0.56	0.57
Depressions					
Salford East	1.46	1.77	1.25	1.30	1.64
Salford West	–	–	1.09	1.12	1.23
Dementias					
Salford East	0.16	0.17	0.26	0.53	0.94
Salford West	–	–	0.35	0.44	0.92
Other neuroses					
Salford East	0.33	0.24	0.22	0.34	0.20
Salford West	–	–	0.25	0.22	0.23
Personality disorders					
Salford East	0.35	0.56	0.54	0.57	0.64
Salford West	–	–	0.17	0.18	0.21
Alcohol and addictions					
Salford East	0.18	0.31	0.31	0.36	0.71
Salford West	–	–	0.18	0.19	0.37
Others					
Salford East	0.25	0.54	0.43	0.54	1.47
Salford West	–	–	0.42	0.41	0.67
Total					
Salford East	4.11	4.63	4.02	4.67	6.55
Salford West	–	–	2.98	3.11	4.20

for young women were always low. In the age group 45–64 years, there has been little change in the last ten years. Above age 65, rates have been increasing, and elderly women increasingly dominate the service. At 1 January 1986, the ten-year accumulation of new long-stay in-patients aged 65 and over was 16 men (3.1 per 1000) and 47 women (5.2 per 1000) from Salford East, and 18 men (1.9 per 1000) and 52 women (3.4 per 1000) from Salford West (Fryers, 1974, 1979*b*).

In spite of rates for Salford West being generally lower, those for the whole city are high and rising. Thus long-stay in-patient care increasingly reflects the domination, in our populations, of health care problems in old age, especially in women. The mental hospital provides most of this care; this is unsatisfactory for patients, and adds to the difficulties of planning its replacement by more appropriate accommodation.

Table 28 gives admission rates for diagnostic groups in Salford East and Salford West. Admissions for schizophrenia have been stable but from Salford East at almost twice the rate of Salford West, directly reflecting the inception data. Depressions are perhaps slightly rising, but there is no doubt about the increase in dementias from both communities, at similar levels. Other neuroses have been stable, but the increase in 'other' diagnoses may well overlap with this group. There have been slight rises in personality disorders, and marked rises in admissions for alcohol-related and other drug-related disorders. Both these groups are admitted about twice as frequently in Salford East as Salford West, again reflecting the difference in inceptions.

The total admission rates have increased substantially only in the latter years of the study, as was seen also in Table 25. In 1986 they were 6.6 per 1000 total population from Salford East, and 4.2 per 1000 from Salford West. The differences in total and in diagnostic distribution presumably reflect differences in socio-economic status, social environments, especially housing, and provision of community resources. It may also reflect some of the specifically 'inner-city' problems characteristic of parts of Salford East. Statistics for electoral wards within the city show considerable variation in admission rates, with the highest three times that of the lowest. The pattern is surprisingly clear; the nearer the area is to the centre of the conurbation, the higher the admission rates for mental illness (Freeman & Alpert, 1986).

Thus there is little evidence that the very considerable extensions of 'community' services in the last two decades have materially affected the use of in-patient care: they have not reduced admissions, not changed the distribution of length of stay, and not reduced the numbers of people admitted for at least a year. They may have affected the balance of diagnostic categories in the admissions rates. More people with schizophrenia are being maintained out of hospital, but more people with dementias, addictions and personality disorders are being admitted instead. Most people would agree that hospital admission, especially prolonged admission, has only a small part to play in the total treatment, rehabilitation, care and support required by most of those receiving these diagnostic labels and in Salford, as elsewhere, current developments are trying to provide more appropriate services. The register may be able to demonstrate the results in a few more years.

Day services

Day care is very complex and difficult to monitor and evaluate. Attendance is very variable in both intensity and duration: functions include therapy, rehabilitation, education, work, occupation, leisure, companionship, and relief of families; purposes of referral are often unclear; and many day facilities are not designated 'mental health' and are therefore not included in the information system. Some of these characteristics may well indicate a 'good' service, but they limit the activities of the register, which routinely collects only episodes of care, not actual attendances, and only from designated specialist facilities, not generic ones. Routine data merely indicate the growth of specialist day care, especially in the health service, which now provides more places than local authority specialist centres. Further information has required special surveys, and cohort studies based on the register.

Two unpublished studies by Cheadle and Fryers have revealed more detail about clients and the full extent of day care for mental illness in Salford. Two cohorts were followed up for four years. One was of all inceptors in 1978 to in-patient care with no previous day-patient experience, and the other was all inceptors in 1978 to day-patient care with no previous in-patient experience. The cohorts were of similar sex distribution, but the day-care group was slightly younger. Those in the in-patient group had more schizophrenia and dementia, but their outstanding feature was that many of them lived alone, and these were mostly elderly, widowed women. It seems that selection by psychiatrists for day care was inhibited by lack of family support, which suggests that support by community nurses or social workers from the point of inception might reduce admissions to hospital.

The day-care cohort had more mild and moderate depressions, but similar numbers of severe depressions to the other cohort. In four years of follow-up there were not large differences between further use of services, and only about 30% of each cohort had any registered mental health service contact during the fourth year. But far more of the in-patient group died, 12% in one year and 23% in four years, compared with none and 10% of the day-care group. This is to some extent related to age, but needs further study. From earlier register studies there is some evidence that admission to a psychiatric bed in old age is related to early death, independent of diagnosis.

In September 1982 there were only four special mental health units, with 203 people attending during the month. There were 15 other 'community units', run by either the local authority or a voluntary agency (e.g. a local church), with 1412 people attending, of whom 167 (12%) were on the psychiatric register, 70 being in current contact. A total month prevalence would be 1.78 per 1000 total population, or 2.41 per 1000 if all registered people are included. Attendance at the mental health centres was quite intense, at an average of 14 out of 22 available days. It was impossible to estimate attendance at most of the community centres as they were often informal, with people coming as and when they pleased, and complete records were not kept.

There were far more centres in Salford East than West, and this excess of provision may well be a reasonable response of the various agencies concerned to greater perceived need in the inner city. The mental health units catered mostly for people in the middle-aged groups, and most elderly people were in the non-specialist community units. This is not unexpected, since distinctions between various health problems and needs in old age are often blurred and of doubtful validity. In these centres over 54% of women were over 65 years old, as were over 30% of men. The corresponding figures for mental health units were 26% and 8%. In both types of centre depressions predominated. Schizophrenia was more common in specialist units, and organic conditions and neuroses more common in the others.

Since those studies, day care has continued to expand. Although the numbers receiving formal mental health day care at any one time are similar in the two communities, the point-prevalence rates are much higher in Salford East, at 1.42 per 1000 total population as of 1 January 1987, than Salford West, at 1.05 per 1000. For the whole of Salford the figure is 1.2 per 1000. We can assume that informal non-specialist day care has also continued to expand. In general, day-care facilities giving social support to mentally ill people, often 'on demand', and integrated into general community provision, have flourished in Salford. But there is little evidence upon which to base any formal evaluation or future plans.

Out-patient services

Attendances, persons attending and population rates for psychiatric out-patient clinics have generally risen since 1976. The number of attendances rose more than the number of people attending, so that the mean annual number of attendances per person increased. Even so, this has been consistently rather less than 3 in recent years, illustrating the large number of people coming to out-patient clinics only once in a year, and who balance the few who attend frequently and regularly for long periods. In 1981, 2454 people (12.6 per 1000 adults) attended 7070 times to see a psychiatrist. In the latest years for which figures are available (1984, 1985) the out-patient rates (per 1000 adults) were 17 per 1000 persons and 45 per 1000 attendances. These figures exclude the 'injection only' visits to a nurse, although these often take place at the same clinics.

'Depressions' is the largest diagnostic group seen in out-patients, accounting for 40% of all attendances. 'Schizophrenias' and 'other neuroses' were next most frequent, but with less than 20% each. The proportion of out-patients given a diagnosis of schizophrenia has been slowly increasing; neuroses have been slowly diminishing. Consistent with all other statistics of service use in Salford, the numbers of people attending out-patients with dementias, and alcohol- and drug-related disorders, have been increasing, especially the latter group. As with other measures, out-patient attendances are considerably higher from the inner-city area, Salford East.

The increasing use of depot neuroleptic drugs in the early 1970s led to the introduction of an 'injection only' out-patient service, in which patients only saw the nurse. These are recorded separately by the register, and have increased very considerably since 1973. Few young or old people attend, and most have a diagnosis of schizophrenia, but in the middle-aged groups, rates of over 2 per 1000 on each annual census have a major impact on the service statistics as a whole.

The register records not only all individual out-patient-type contacts, but also the site of those contacts. Well over half take place at the general hospital psychiatric unit where numbers have not changed recently. But people seen at the large mental hospital have decreased considerably, while those seen at general practice health centres and other community bases scattered throughout the city increased from 81 (168 attendances) in 1976 to 279 (850 attendances) in 1981, and has continued to increase since. For 1985 the distribution was: hospital out-patients 6308; community-service bases, 1314; visits at home, 836; consultations on general hospital wards, 211; others, 15.

This documents the increasing diversity and dispersion of the service and, one hopes, increasing convenience for patients and efficiency of operation. But there is a danger in the loss to the mental hospital of out-patient care as well as short-stay in-patient care, if it becomes merely the repository for failures. This points to the need to develop policies directly concerned with alternatives to long-stay care in the mental hospital, if it is not to have its institutional disadvantages and reputation reinforced, and if it is ever going to be replaced by more suitable facilities.

Community psychiatric nursing

The community psychiatric nursing service in Salford (see Chapter 6) was in large part a response to the potential for maintaining people with schizophrenia in their own homes with the help of depot neuroleptic drugs, and the need for supervision and support which this implied. It has other attractions, however; it both extends the options of care for all individual patients in a less stigmatising, more 'ordinary life' setting, and offers more independence and job satisfaction to the nurses. From its inception in 1973, it grew very rapidly in a somewhat unplanned and haphazard way. From three nurses working from the mental hospital following up patients who failed to attend out-patient clinics, it grew to 18 nurses by October 1982, all attached to general practitioners, and all receiving direct referrals without recourse to psychiatrists.

The statistics of the service reveal the expansion, monitored since the beginning of 1976 by a major study (Wooff *et al*, 1986). The one-day prevalence for all current contacts with the nurses, whether or not patients were also in contact with other parts of the service, rose progressively from 0.4 per 1000 adults in 1976 to 6.8 per 1000 adults at the beginning of 1985. The year prevalence figures rose from 1.5 per 1000 in 1976 to 11.8 per 1000 adults in 1985. The numbers in only recent contact, the equivalent of 'short-term care', have remained very small, but by 1983 over half the total on the census had been in continuous care of the community nurses for over a year, mostly over two years. Thus the community nurses have been steadily accumulating their own 'long-stay cases'.

Although originally concentrating on people with schizophrenia, once the new service was established it rapidly extended to all other diagnostic groups. In particular, even by 1979 more people with depression were seen in the year (year prevalence) than with schizophrenia, who constituted under 23% of the whole at 2.0 per 1000 adults. By 1982, the distribution of diagnoses in the community nursing service had become almost identical to that in the mental health services as a whole.

Similarly, relatively few elderly people were visited by the first community psychiatric nurses, but by 1982 the over 75 age group gave the highest year prevalence rates, and the age distribution for community nursing was similar to the mental health services as a whole. At the same time, more people, especially with depressions, have been retained under community nurse care without other contacts within the year. In the point-prevalence figures, a majority of their patients in every diagnostic group received no other mental health care. It should be remembered, however, that the nurses are working from general practice health centres and might be viewed as a specialist arm of general practice just as much as a domiciliary arm of the psychiatric service.

We have already seen that contacts with psychiatrists, admissions and even long-stay in-patient care have not diminished in the period of the rise of the new community nursing service, and similarly, there has been no decrease in specialist mental health social work. Thus community nurses have in no way substituted for psychiatrists or social workers. It is unlikely that they have taken more referrals from psychiatrists to supplement their care for the same patients, as they have become very independent of the psychiatrists, and have many exclusive patients.

As the new service seems largely to have added cases to the total receiving definable 'mental health' care, it seems likely that they have gained most of their case loads from those previously receiving mainly general practice support. The register is not able to record any effect this might have had on the work of general practitioners, but its impact on the statistics of the rest of the mental health service seems to have been minimal (Wooff et al, 1986; Wooff, 1987).

Mental health social work

Mental health social work has a special history in Salford, and is a peculiar feature of the Salford register (Wooff, 1978; Freeman, 1979). In the 1960s a large group of professional, specialist social workers was built up by the local authority of Salford East (Susser, 1968). They worked in close association with both hospital psychiatrists and general practitioners. In 1971 a new generic social services department took over all social work, and both the specialist mental health service and the close working contact with doctors were lost. Some social workers became attached to hospitals for liaison, and these eventually established a *de facto* specialist mental health social work service again. It is ironic that they are based at hospitals, although employed by the local authority, whereas the previous service was wholly community based.

The statistics describe this history and the interaction of social work with other parts of the service (Wooff et al, 1983). In Salford East in 1969, the point prevalence for mental health social work was 2.18 per 1000 adults, but this diminished considerably after reorganisation of the services and the loss of specialists. This was not merely a recording problem; the register continued to record all contacts with generic social workers that involved a 'mental health' problem. Changes of definition were inevitable, but even on the verifiable definition of 'currently in contact with a psychiatrist', numbers diminished considerably (Wooff, 1978). By 1976 numbers were back to the 1968 levels as the specialist service was re-established, although 25% of contacts were with generic 'area team' social workers.

By this time, community psychiatric nurses were invading the scene in increasing numbers, working especially with people with schizophrenia, which had been the principal emphasis of the social work service in 1968. The distribution of diagnoses in social work contacts concurrently shifted to more people with depressions and then other diagnoses, and more elderly people. By 1979 both domiciliary services (nursing and social work) carried similar numbers of people, and adding together the census figures gave 4.66 per 1000 adults, prevalence rates more than double the rates for 1969.

Before amalgamation in 1974, mental health social work was not strong in Salford West, but since then the service there has also built up. Not surprisingly in the light of all the other statistics distinguishing the two communities, mental health social work is much more extensively used in Salford East, the inner-city area. Since 1982, day-prevalence rates, which represent case loads, have been running at about 1 per 1000 adults in the West and 2 per 1000 in the East. Inceptions have also been different, at 1.5 per 1000 and 2 per 1000 respectively in 1982, and total referrals were 2.6 per 1000 and 4.2 per 1000. In both communities inceptions are higher in the over 75 age group. In Salford as a whole, by 1986 total annual referrals were over 5 per 1000 adults, with higher rates for those aged 65–74 years, and even higher for those aged 75 and over. The point prevalence for 1 January 1985 was 2.5 per 1000 adults, and the year prevalence for 1985 was 8.0 per 1000.

In recent years, approximately 35% of referrals were for 'depression', about 20% for schizophrenia (more in Salford East), and about 12% each for 'other neuroses' and personality disorders. Alcohol- and drug-related disorders and dementias have both increased to over 5%. About 20% of case loads were people of very recent contact, but about 40% had been retained on a case load for over one year, mostly over two years.

For many years, the evidence suggested that mental health social workers and community psychiatric nurses provided very similar services in statistical terms. They were of similar size, served a similar mix of people in terms of age and diagnosis, and retained cases for very similar periods of support. However, in the last few years community nursing has continued to increase its case load numbers, which now give point-prevalence figures almost three times those for social work, although only 1.5 times the year prevalence. There are some obvious differences in tasks; for example, only nurses may give injections, and only social workers are likely to be able to negotiate their way through welfare benefit regulations, but these hardly constitute significant professional differences, and do not reflect their almost totally different selection, training, traditions and circumstances of employment. The ways in which they perceive their roles and the way in which they perform their work are also very different. These and other differences are explored in Wooff's (1987) study of the two groups in Salford.

Summary and conclusions

The psychiatric register has monitored all contacts with a comprehensive range of mental health services from a defined, diminishing, inner-city population since 1968, and an additional suburban population since 1975. Data are collected systematically in standard form and stored in cumulative, individual records on computer. Routine analysis includes annual point prevalence, inceptions, admissions, cohort follow-up, etc.

Annual census totals have increased considerably since 1978, particularly for depressions and dementias of old age, in women more than men, and especially for disorders related to alcohol and drugs. Increases in numbers of both patients in contact and annual contacts per patient resulted in period prevalence increases also. These changes reflect the progressive addition of new services.

Inceptions (totally new cases) changed little between ages of 45 and 64 years, decreased at lower ages, and increased fairly dramatically at higher ages. There were generally higher rates in the inner city compared with the suburbs, especially for alcohol, drug, and personality disorders, and for younger women. Much greater demand for mental health care arises in the parts of Salford that have experienced more disruption of communities and more social problems. Compared with the inner city, there are far fewer admissions to hospital from the suburbs in all diagnostic groups, and for small areas, the closer to the city centre, the higher the admission rates. Admissions to hospital, number of persons admitted, and residents of under three months' stay (all mostly at the general hospital), have all varied very little. Numbers of in-patients with lengths of stay between one and ten years have been generally stable in middle age, falling for young adults and rising for elderly people. Numbers staying over ten years have been falling, mostly by death. The inner city shows much higher long-stay statistics because a dramatic fall in population has affected the denominator.

Day care has increased and become very dispersed, varied, and to a large extent non-specialist. Out-patients have also increased in total and in the variety of contacts. Most contacts are at the general hospital unit; those at the mental hospital are decreasing, while those at health centres are increasing. 'Injection-only' visits to clinics for neuroleptic drugs administered by a nurse make a major contribution, especially to patients with schizophrenia. Community psychiatric nursing has increased dramatically since its inception in 1973 and current contacts show a similar age and diagnostic distribution to the rest of the service. After a fall in the early 1970s, mental health social work also increased as the specialist service was reintroduced.

For the elderly, increasing services are a response to the generally perceived increase in need, although it is doubtful whether they are keeping pace. In general, Salford has expanded mental health services very considerably, representing a large increase in resources. These have mostly increased the care options available to people living 'in the community', yet they have not resulted in significant reductions in in-patient or psychiatric hospital care. If this is to be effected, it will require a deliberate policy of diminution, as part of a comprehensive community mental health service plan.

This chapter has briefly surveyed the various basic measures that a register can provide to monitor a community mental health service, and so revealed a host of conflicts in the current and changing situation in Salford. It would be too simplistic to offer conclusions beyond the most general; many of the details raise interesting, important and difficult issues in themselves. But several general impressions are hard to avoid.

Group homes have been established, day care has become diversified and less specialised, out-patients have increasingly been seen in primary care health centres, many patients are maintained at home on depot drugs, social workers are again offering a specialist service, and numbers of community psychiatric nurses have burgeoned. Yet the effect on the traditional hospital services has been surprisingly small; conventional out-patients and specialist day care have increased, and admission rates and lengths of in-patient stay have not fallen. Indeed some have risen, particularly for elderly people. This has important implications for other communities in the process of 'developing' mental health services.

Certainly the increasing number of old people, and particularly the very old, is a real and no doubt lasting phenomenon, and the establishment of a specialist psychogeriatric service, which concentrates great effort on assessment at home, rehabilitation and avoidance of admission wherever possible, is having an increasing impact. But in what other ways the increasing amount of mental health care in Salford represents previous 'unmet need' is difficult to judge. It is possible that such 'need' is virtually limitless, but there must be limits on the resources made available. Uncontrolled expansion may not in the end be the best way of achieving a satisfactory, comprehensive, high-quality service. It is easier to reduce the number of community nurses than not to staff a mental hospital ward if the economic crunch comes!

The types of people admitted to in-patient care have changed since 1976. Is this also unmet need, or is it merely the inevitable tendency to fill 'beds' which exist, with all their ancillary resources? The expansion of community support services, however good in itself, will not necessarily result in reduction in hospital care. If this is to happen, positive policies have to be agreed, and definitive plans have to be implemented progressively to reduce the mental hospital at the same time as building up alternative services. This needs to be done for two reasons: to release the resources of money, skills and personnel for better use, and to provide more humane, civilised and dignified forms of care for mentally ill people in the future.

Acknowledgements

This chapter is up-dated, modified and expanded from "Monitoring mental health services in an English city", a chapter published in Italian in Tansella (1985). Thanks are due to Malcolm Cleverly for computing, and Paul Fryers for preparation of the tables. The Salford Mental Health Information Unit is supported by Salford District Health Authority and Salford Department of Social Services.

References

ADELSTEIN, A. M., DOWNHAM, D. Y., STEIN, Z., *et al* (1968) The epidemiology of mental illness in an English city. *Social Psychiatry*, **3**, 47–49.

FREEMAN, H. L. (1979) *The History of Mental Health Services in Salford*. MSc thesis, University of Salford.

—— & ALPERT, M. (1986) Prevalence of schizophrenia: geographical variations in an urban population. *British Journal of Social and Clinical Psychology*, **4**, 67–75.

FRYERS, T. (1974) Psychiatric in-patients in 1982: how many beds? *Psychological Medicine*, **4**, 196–211.

—— (1976a) Psychiatric service planning; beds in perspective. *Comprehensive Psychiatry*, **7**, 361–368.

—— (1976b) Mental health services: statistics and policy. *International Journal of Mental Health*, **5**, 14–21.

—— (1979a) Estimation of need on the basis of case register studies: British case register data. In *Estimating Needs for Mental Health Care* (ed. H. Häfner). Berlin: Springer-Verlag.

—— (1979b) Accumulating long stay in-patients in Salford: monitoring further progress. *Psychological Medicine*, **9**, 567–572.

—— (1986a) Use of the Salford psychiatric register for administrative and operational research. In *The Use of Psychiatric Case Registers in Public Health, 1960–1985* (eds G. H. M. ten Horn *et al*), pp. 101–114. Amsterdam: Elsevier.

—— (1986b) Practical issues in the establishment, maintenance, and exploitation of registers; Introduction. In *The Use of Psychiatric Case Registers in Public Health, 1960–1985* (eds G. H. M. M. ten Horn *et al*), pp. 262–268. Amsterdam: Elsevier.

——, FREEMAN, H. L. & MOUNTNEY, G. H. (1970) A census of psychiatric patients in an urban community. *Social Psychiatry*, **5**, 187–193.

GIBBONS, J., JENNINGS, C. & WING, J. K. (1984) *Psychiatric Care in Eight Register Areas*. Southampton: University Department of Psychiatry. (Copies obtainable by sending £2.50, cheque payable to University of Southampton, to University Department of Psychiatry, Royal South Hants Hospital, Southampton SO9 4PE.)

MOUNTNEY, G. H., FRYERS, T. & FREEMAN, H. L. (1969) Psychiatric emergencies in an urban borough. *British Medical Journal*, *i*, 498–500.

SUSSER, M. W. (1968) *Community Psychiatry: Epidemiologic and Social Themes*. New York: Random House.

——, STEIN, Z., MOUNTNEY, G. H., *et al* (1969) Chronic disability following mental illness in an English city: part I. *Social Psychiatry*, **4**, 82–91.

——, ——, ——, *et al* (1970) Chronic disability following mental illness in an English city: part II. *Social Psychiatry*, **5**, 69–76.

TANSELLA, M. (1985) *L'Approccio Epidemiologico in Psichiatria*. Turin: Boringhien.

WING, J. K. & HAILEY, A. M. (eds) (1972) *Evaluating a Community Psychiatric Service*. Oxford: Oxford University Press.

—— & FRYERS, T. (1976) *Psychiatric Services in Camberwell and Salford: Statistics from the Camberwell and Salford Case Registers, 1964–1974*. Vol. 1, pp. 1–100, comparative statistics; Vol. 2, pp. 101–140, appendices and bibliography. Institute of Psychiatry, University of London, and Department of Community Medicine, University of Manchester.

WING, L. (1970) Observations on the psychiatric section of the International Classification of Diseases, and the British Glossary of Mental Disorders. *Psychological Medicine*, **1**, 79–85.

WOOFF, K. (1978) *The Use of Social Services by Psychiatric Patients in Salford*. MSc thesis, University of Manchester.

—— (1987) *A Comparison of the Work of Community Psychiatric Nurses and Mental Health Social Workers in Salford*. PhD thesis, University of Manchester.

——, FREEMAN, H. L. & FRYERS, T. (1983) Psychiatric service use in Salford C.B.: a comparison of point prevalence ratios 1968 and 1978. *British Journal of Psychiatry*, **142**, 588–597.

——, GOLDBERG, D. P. & FRYERS, T. (1986) Patients in receipt of community psychiatric nursing care in Salford, 1976–1982. *Psychological Medicine*, **16**, 407–414.

4 The effects of population changes on long-stay in-patient rates

G. DER

The demographic and social differences between register areas are described by Gibbons *et al* (1984) and are summarised in Chapter 1. The marked differences in the rates of bed occupancy (particularly for very-long-stay in-patients) shown in Chapter 2 cannot be interpreted without further analysis of the point prevalence rates used.

McMahon & Pugh (1970) point out that:

> "three items of information are necessary for a rate to have epidemiologic usefulness – the numerator of the fraction (the number of persons affected), the denominator (the population among whom the affected persons are observed), and a specification of time . . . for a specified population at a specified time, point prevalence rate is the proportion of that population which exhibits the disease at that particular time. The numerator includes all persons having the disease at the given moment, irrespective of the length of time which has elapsed from the beginning of the illness to the time when the point prevalence is measured. The denominator is the total population (affected and unaffected) within which the disease is ascertained."

In common with other descriptive statistics, the point prevalence rate is more applicable to some situations than others, and using it inappropriately may lead to statistical artefacts and false comparisons. If the length of time from the beginning of the disorder to the prevalence point is great enough, the population may have changed in the meantime. When this period extends to 60 years (and in Camberwell, Nottingham and Worcester about 1% of in-patients had been resident for longer than this), it is evident that the base population could well have changed markedly.

Changes in population size

In order to provide comparable rates, registers require a geographically defined population base. The population included by such a definition varies over time, both because of changing patterns of births and deaths, and because of migration into and out of the area.

High levels of net emigration are often associated with an overall decline in the prosperity of the area in question. This is most obvious in areas dependent on one or more forms of industry, such as coal mining or ship building, that are in decline. In such cases the resultant emigration may leave behind a population containing a higher proportion of the old, poor and chronically ill. A similar tendency can be found in some inner-city areas, but the causes and results are more complex. If migration is selective in this way, it may lead to increased or decreased levels of morbidity in the base population, and hence to differences in rates of disorder. Part of these differences could be due simply to a change in population size, and it is important to distinguish this from changes in social and demographic constitution.

Register data

Figure 1 (p. 6) shows the relative change in population size for seven register areas since 1921. Assuming the curve for England indicates the average change due to birth and death rates, high levels of net migration are evident in four of the areas.

Table 29 shows the in-patient prevalence rates for eight register areas in three broad length-of-stay groups, namely: under one year ('short-stay'), one to five years ('medium-long-stay') and five years or more ('very-long-stay'). Large differences between the areas are evident in each of the length-of-stay groups.

The main concern here is with the very-long-stay group, since the effect of population change is minimal on shorter lengths of stay. It is notable that in the very-long-stay group there are high rates in Camberwell and Salford, the two areas that have had marked population decline, and low rates in the two areas where most increase has occurred – Oxford and Worcester. This suggests the hypothesis that the population change itself has contributed to the difference in rates, whether through differential migration or in virtue of the way in which the statistic is calculated. This could not be the whole explanation, since Aberdeen has the highest rate but has not undergone a population decline like that in Camberwell and Salford. Moreover, the Scottish rate for the very-long-stay is twice that of England and Wales, suggesting that the explanation for a high rate in Aberdeen is likely to depend on factors specific to Scotland.

Aberdeen, Camberwell and Salford also have high rates in the short-stay and medium-long-stay groups, while Oxford and Worcester have low rates. In the short-stay group, the high rates in Camberwell and Aberdeen correspond to a

TABLE 29
Resident in-patients at 31 December 1981 – rates per 100 000 population

Area	Under 1 year	1 < 5 years	5 years and over	Total
Aberdeen	102	70	110	283
Camberwell	126	54	89	271
Cardiff	63	46	60	169
Nottingham	68	41	51	160
Oxford	39	16	20	75
Salford	71	59	108	238
Southampton	73	35	38	145
Worcester	40	20	35	94
England	58	38	62	156
Wales	57	34	64	155
Scotland	87	82	136	305

high admission rate (see Chapter 2) and are probably explained by the availability of extra beds.

Correcting for change in population size

Persons admitted to hospital can be regarded as representative only of the population at the time they were admitted. Correcting subsequent rates to allow for any changes in population size is done by differentially weighting the contribution of each in-patient to the overall prevalence according to the size of population at the time he/she was admitted. Each in-patient is counted as the reciprocal of the population at the time of admission and the corrected rate is formed from the sum of these numbers. If no change in population size has occurred, the contribution of each in-patient will be the same and the rate will be exactly the same. If the population has halved during a given period, those admitted at the beginning of that period will contribute only half as much towards the total.

It is impractical to estimate the population of the area for each date on which a resident in-patient was admitted, especially as the main source of population data is likely to be the ten-yearly national censuses. Instead, calculations are made to the nearest whole year; equivalent to calculating separate rates for each group of resident in patients who were admitted in the same year, using the population of the register area in that year, and summing the separate rates. Briefly the procedure is as follows.

(a) The number of patients in hospital is broken down by the length of stay in whole years.
(b) The length of stay is then subtracted from the year of the prevalence point to give a breakdown by year of admission (this would not be strictly accurate if the prevalence point were not the end of the year).
(c) The figures for each year are then turned into rates based on the population of the area during that year.
(d) These separate rates are summed to form the overall rate.

The prevalence point chosen was the end of 1981. Each of the eight registers supplied a breakdown of the numbers of in-patients at that point by length of stay in whole years (not rounded to the nearest year). Length of stay was calculated on the basis of continuous residence in psychiatric hospitals. As far as possible transfers between psychiatric hospitals were not counted as discharges. This was relatively unproblematic for transfers which had occurred since the register had begun and were therefore recorded on the register routinely. However, registers differed in their treatment of transfers that had been made prior to the commencement of the register.

When a register is set up, information is collected on all the in-patients resident at the time, but the registers differed as to what they treated as the date of admission for those in-patients. Camberwell and Salford recorded previous transfers and attempted to trace back to the original admission. Most other registers took the date of admission of the current spell.

In theory this is an important difference between registers, since an unrecorded transfer will have the effect of artificially shortening the length of stay and thereby affecting the amount of adjustment that should be made. On the other hand, a number of register areas contained relatively few psychiatric hospitals and transfers between them were rare.

Estimates of the base population for each register area for each year in which any of the resident in-patients were admitted were obtained by making a linear projection between the two nearest censuses, unless the year was itself a census year, in which case the census figure was used. As can be seen from Fig. 1, the population trends between 1921 and 1981 in most cases contained few marked peaks or troughs. The shape of the population curve would not matter if the length of stay could be assumed to have been accurately ascertained. The fact that there is a steady trend becomes important if there are a significant number of unrecorded transfers. It implies that the adjustment will be conservative, in that it will underestimate the amount of correction which would have been necessary had the length of stay been measured accurately.

Results

Table 30 presents the results of the adjustment on the rates of very-long-stay in-patients alongside the crude rates given in Table 29.

The overall effect of the adjustment has been to reduce the differences between registers, as well as those between registers and their respective national figures. For instance, the rate for Aberdeen moves closer to that for all Scotland. Without adjustment or comparison with the national rates the Aberdeen and Salford rates might have appeared similar. This apparent similarity is clearly an artefact. So too is the apparently high rate in Camberwell relative to that of England.

As the population of England has increased by 30% since 1921, the English national rate should also be adjusted for strict comparability. (The Scottish population only increased by 4% in the same period.) However, the national figures are not available in sufficient detail for the adjustment to be made. An alternative would be to make a second adjustment to the registers' rates to correct for the national population change. This has not been done here, but when applied to the Camberwell figures it resulted in a further decrease in the rate by 13% relative to that of England (Wing & Der, 1984).

TABLE 30

Long-stay in-patients over five years at 31 December 1981 – rates per 100 000 population

Area	Crude rate	Adjusted rate
Aberdeen	110	119
Camberwell	89	60
Cardiff	60	60
Nottingham	51	50
Oxford	20	29
Salford	108	88
Southampton	38	38
Worcester	35	43
England	62	–
Wales	64	–
Scotland	136	–

It is also clear that the correction by no means removes all the differences in the rates, and there are still marked differences between the register areas. For the reasons mentioned above, the correction may be an underestimate. Nonetheless, removing some of the differences helps to clarify the comparison. It is also unlikely that the remaining differences are due solely to the treatment of transfers.

Population change may still be an important factor in the sense already mentioned, that migration may have been selective of people more or less prone to mental illness. Oxford and Worcester are obviously very different areas from Camberwell and Salford, being relatively prosperous mixed rural and urban areas, while the latter are inner-city areas in large conurbations. On a range of socio-demographic indicators drawn from the 1981 census for the eight register areas, Camberwell and Salford are the two worst off, and Oxford and Worcester the two most privileged. These factors are likely to have affected admission rates differentially.

Giggs (1984), who reviewed the work on residential mobility and mental health, concluded:

> "It is probably the case, therefore, that high inner city admission rates are the product of a combination of local socially vulnerable and disorganised populations (the breeder hypothesis), the inward movement of similar individuals (the drift hypothesis), and the selective outward movement of those healthy individuals who are both willing and able to do so (the social residue hypothesis)."

Hospital residents at any point in time represent an accumulation from admissions over a long period, and so the explanation of high rates is likely to be even more complex. Moreover, the relative balance of the three factors might well have changed over such a period.

Although this paper has focused on technical aspects, there are also important practical implications. Inner-city areas with high admission rates, both past and present, but with unexceptional rates of recruitment to long-stay in-patient status from these admissions, would end up with high long-stay in-patient rates. If, in addition, they had undergone marked population decline, as is typical of such areas, their rates would appear even higher. Conversely, rural and green-belt areas with equivalent levels of population increase could expect to have correspondingly low rates. A policy of funding health districts according to the current size of their catchment area, and expecting all to conform to an overall national average, would be a classic case of giving to those that have and taking from those that have not.

References

GIBBONS, J., JENNINGS, C. & WING, J. K. (1984) *Psychiatric Care in Eight Register Areas.* Southampton: University Department of Psychiatry. (Copies obtainable by sending £2.50, cheque payable to University of Southampton, to University Department of Psychiatry, Royal South Hants Hospital, Southampton SO9 4PE.)

GIGGS, J. A. (1984) Residential mobility and mental health. In *Mental Health and the Environment* (ed. H. L. Freeman). London: Churchill Livingstone.

McMAHON, B. & PUGH, T. F. (1970) *Epidemiology: Principles and Methods.* Boston: Little, Brown.

WING, J. K. & DER, G. (1984) *Report of the Camberwell Register 1980–1984.* London: MRC Social Psychiatry Unit.

5 Powick Hospital, 1978–86: a case register study

C. HASSALL and S. ROSE

The Worcester Development Project, funded by the Department of Health and Social Security, was designed to replace a system of mental health care centred on an old mental hospital (Powick Hospital near Worcester) with a community-based psychiatric service. The new service is characterised by the provision of facilities in the main population centres of the catchment area (Department of Health and Social Security, 1970; Hassall, 1976), which comprises most of the old county of Worcestershire. The facilities provided under the project are shown in Table 31. Central to the project was the opening of two new psychiatric in-patient units sited in Worcester and Kidderminster: once these were opened it was planned that Powick would be closed to admissions.

The feasibility study (Department of Health and Social Security, 1970), made in 1968, envisaged that Powick would cease to admit patients in 1973. In 1980, when it was predicted that only 250 patients would remain, the hospital would close. The study recommended that, "By 1975 the Regional Hospital Board and Hospital Management Committee will need to complete plans for the disposal of remaining patients to a selected hospital in the neighbourhood". The delays, inevitable in a project of this scale, were such that the two new in-patient units were not opened until July (Kidderminster) and December (Worcester) 1978. Thus from the end of 1978, with 343 patients in residence, Powick Hospital was closed to admissions.

TABLE 31
Worcester Development Project

Unit	Area	Opening date
Psychiatric hostel	Kidderminster	1 July 1976
Day centre	Malvern	17 January 1977
Day centre	Worcester	17 January 1977
Psychiatric in-patient unit and day hospital	Kidderminster	3 July 1978
Psychiatric in-patient unit and day hospital	Newtown–Worcester	6 December 1978
Day hospital	Malvern	19 February 1979
Day hospital	Evesham	2 March 1979
Day centre	Droitwich	18 April 1979
Day centre	Kidderminster	18 June 1979
Alcoholism in-patient unit and day hospital	Newtown–Worcester	12 February 1979 14 May 1979
Unit for elderly people with psychiatric disorders	Newtown–Worcester	1 September 1983

It has not proved possible to transfer the remaining patients to a neighbouring hospital, as most have their own quota of long-term residents and are keen to use any free wards to enhance their own resources. At the end of 1986 therefore Powick was still open and the home of 114 long-stay patients. The problems of running a hospital where there are no admissions and very few discharges have been dealt with elsewhere (Gillard, 1984; Hassall & Cross, 1979; Markwick, 1980). This chapter examines the attrition of the population remaining in the hospital at the end of 1978 and the experience of those who were discharged.

Method

Using the case register it is possible to determine the deaths in Powick and the use of the psychiatric services by those who were discharged. As the register does not cover part-3 homes or other local authority sheltered accommodation, information about those discharged to this type of care had to be obtained directly from staff in contact with the patients.

Results

The census populations 1978 and 1986

At the end of 1978 when Powick was closed to admissions there were 343 patients in residence. The most important features of this population, in terms of the

TABLE 32

Powick Hospital census population 31 December 1978 and 31 December 1986, by age group

Age group	Males		Females		Total	
	1978	*1986*	*1978*	*1986*	*1978*	*1986*
	(n = 146)	*(n = 53)*	*(n = 197)*	*(n = 61)*	*(n = 343)*	*(n = 114)*
	(%)	*(%)*	*(%)*	*(%)*	*(%)*	*(%)*
<45	8	4	2	–	4	2
45<65	38	51	18	20	27	34
65<75	29	24	33	15	31	19
75<85	20	13	31	39	27	27
85 and over	5	8	16	26	11	18

TABLE 33

Powick Hospital census populations 31 December 1978 and 31 December 1986, by diagnostic group and length of stay

	1978 (n = 343) (%)	*1986* (n = 114) (%)
Diagnostic groups		
All dementia	15	8
Schizophrenia and all other psychoses	71	74
Neurosis, personality disorders, depression, and alcoholism	3	6
Mental retardation	8	12
Other	3	–
Length of stay		
<10 years	44	16
10–20 years	14	22
20–30 years	11	16
30–40 years	14	16
40 years and over	17	30

possible run down of the hospital, were; first, the age distribution – 69% of the patients being 65 years or more (54% of males and 80% of the females) (Table 32); second, the diagnostic grouping – nearly three-quarters of the patients were suffering from schizophrenia or other psychosis, and a further 15% from dementia; third, the length of stay – 42% of the census population had been in hospital for 20 years or more (Table 33). By the end of 1986 there were 114 patients remaining in hospital. The proportion of males had risen from 43% to 46%; the percentage of patients aged 65 and over had fallen to 64%. When the diagnostic groups are considered, the 'dementia' group has fallen from 15% to 8% of the total (numerically from 52 to 9 patients) and, although there is little difference in the proportion in the 1978 and 1986 populations, those in the 'schizophrenia' group fell in numbers, from 244 to 84 patients. Similarly, whereas the proportion of those with a stay of 20 years or more has increased by 20% between the census years, the number of patients in this category has actually fallen from 144 to 71 patients.

Patients leaving hospital

Table 34 is a summary of those patients leaving hospital in terms of their characteristics of sex, age, diagnosis and length of stay as at the end of 1978.

TABLE 34
Characteristics of patients who left hospital, as at 31 December 1978

	Died	Transferred	Discharged	Total leaving	% leaving
Sex					
male	79	4	10	93	64
(n = 146)					
female	102	14	20	136	68
(n = 197)					
Age group					
65 years or less	28	5	13	46	43
(n = 107)					
65–75 years	57	6	10	73	69
(n = 105)					
75–85 years	67	5	6	78	84
(n = 93)					
85 years and over	29	2	1	32	84
(n = 38)					
Diagnostic group					
dementia	36	2	5	43	83
(n = 52)					
schizophrenia or	135	15	20	170	70
other psychosis					
(n = 244)					
mentally retarded	9	–	4	13	48
(n = 27)					
other	2	–	1	3	15
(n = 20)					
Length of stay					
10 years or less	122	5	15	142	93
(n = 152)					
10–20 years	6	5	5	16	33
(n = 48)					
20 years and over	53	18	10	71	50
(n = 143)					

Thus 64% of the males and 68% of the females left hospital during the eight years under review, mostly by death. The proportion of each age group leaving hospital by death rises (not surprisingly) with age: this is reflected in the overall proportion of patients leaving which shows the same trend. Most of the discharges occurred in patients under the age of 75 years.

As might be expected, the 'dementia' group showed the greatest (proportionate) reduction – 83% of those bearing this diagnosis in the 1978 census left hospital during the eight years, only five persons being discharged. The major diagnostic group, the 'schizophrenia' group, had declined by 70% (170 persons), with 135 of these patients dying.

Patients who had been in hospital for less than ten years when Powick was closed to admissions showed a very high rate of death, accounting for over half the total number of leavers in the whole population.

When the two new in-patient units opened they each received a group of patients transferred from Powick. In March 1979, however, a further group of 15 patients was transferred to Newtown psychiatric unit in Worcester. These transfers had not been planned originally and had for three months formed part of the residual population in Powick; they have therefore been treated as though they had remained in Powick: in fact most of them died in Newtown and all of them had died by the end of 1984.

Deaths, transfers and discharges

The results are summarised in Table 35.

Deaths

During the eight years under review, 181 patients died in Powick; more than half of these deaths occurred in patients who had (in 1978) been in hospital for less than ten years.

TABLE 35
Patients leaving hospital 1979–86

	1979	1980	1981	1982	1983	1984	1985	1986	Total
General hospital	4	1	–	–	–	1	3	3	12
Psychiatric hospital or geriatric ward	1	–	–	1	1	1	–	2	6
Part-3 accommodation	5	1	1	2	2	–	1	–	12
Hostel	3	1	–	–	–	1	–	–	5
Other sheltered	4	–	–	–	–	–	–	–	4
Community	2	2	–	–	–	–	–	–	4
Out of area	1	1	–	–	–	–	–	–	2
Private nursing home	–	–	–	–	–	–	2	–	2
Died	49	29	21	15	24	14	13	16	181
Summary									
died after discharge to hospital	5	1	–	–	–	2	3	3	14
died after discharge to community	6	4	1	2	–	–	1	–	14
still alive	8[1]	1	–	1	2	1	2[1]	3	18[2]

1. Patient left the area and could not be traced.
2. Excluding two patients who left the area and could not be traced.

The largest number of deaths took place in 1979, followed by 1980, and together these two years accounted for 43% of the total deaths occurring between 1978 and 1986.

Transfers

Of the 18 patients who were transferred to other hospitals, 12 went to a general hospital for treatment of physical illness; all of these died in the hospital within a short time of admission. Six patients were transferred to psychiatric hospital (one outside the catchment area) and one went to a geriatric ward. Three of these patients died; the lady who left the catchment area was subsequently discharged to community care, but no current information about her was available.

Discharges

Almost half the discharges took place in 1979. Twenty-four of the patients were discharged to sheltered or protected environments, such as part-3 accommodation (12), hostel (5), a home for the deaf (1), private nursing home (2), housing under the aegis of the adult training centre (2), and supervised lodgings (1).

Four patients could be said to be discharged to the community in the sense that they lived in unsupervised accommodation: three lived in council flats, and one man went home to his wife.

Two patients left the area. One left of his own accord, but since it was felt that he could manage and it was known that he was familiar with and to most of the social service agencies in the surrounding areas, he was formally discharged. Another patient went to Wales on leave, where he died.

Follow-up

It is clear that the length of follow-up varies considerably between patients; however the intention is to describe the service use of a fairly typical group of long-term patients discharged from hospital over eight years (Table 36).

TABLE 36
Discharge destination by location at end of follow-up (31 December 1986)

Discharge destination	Died	Follow-up location						
		Part-3 accom-modation	Sheltered accom-modation	Private nursing home	Psychiatric hospital geriatric ward	Community	Untraced	Other
General hospital	12	–	–	–	–	–	–	–
Part-3 accommodation	7	3	1	1	–	–	–	–
Sheltered accommodation	–	–	2	1	–	–	–	1
Private nursing home	1	–	–	1	–	–	–	–
Community	2	1	–	–	–	1	–	–
Psychiatric hospital or geriatric ward	3	–	–	–	2	–	1	–
Hostel	2	1	–	–	–	1	–	–
Out of area	1	–	–	–	–	–	1	–

The outcome of discharge was unhappy in two cases: one patient committed suicide and another was sent to a special hospital after a conviction for arson; he remains in that hospital. Of the 12 patients who moved to part-3 accommodation, seven died and one was transferred to a private nursing home; three remained in part-3 accommodation. One patient was admitted to the psychiatric unit, where he was reassessed and judged suitable for warden-supervised accommodation, to which he was discharged and where he remains.

Among those who were discharged to hostels, two died, one was the suicide cited above, the other a female patient who stayed for three years before she died. A further patient went on to part-3 accommodation and another to a group home.

The two patients accommodated by the adult training centre left to live in a council flat for two years before taking up residence in warden-supervised housing; one of the two was subsequently admitted to a private nursing home.

One of the patients discharged to a council flat continued to live there for six years until she died: one remained there for almost two years until she took a place in a group home, the third lived in a flat for two years until she had to be admitted to part-3 accommodation. The male patient who went home to his wife became ill after only a few weeks and was admitted to hospital where he died. The patient who lived in a home for the deaf was still there at the end of the follow-up period.

Thus 17 of the discharged patients are known to be still alive at the end of 1986; two could not be traced.

Table 36 shows the accommodation of the patients at the end of 1986; only two were currently in-patients, both on a psychogeriatric ward, although nine of them had spent some time in psychiatric hospital during their follow-up period. Two patients had moved to a less sheltered environment than the one to which they were discharged (from part-3 to sheltered accommodation and from hostel to the community). Two people moved into part-3 accommodation and one to a nursing home.

Service use by discharged patients

Twenty-two patients made use of either the psychiatric services or the local authority services or both after discharge. Tables 37 and 38 show the number of patients using each service each year and the mean number of days per patient using the service. The mean number of in-patient days, particularly in the years 1982, 1985 and 1986, is substantial, but in each of these years only two patients used the service. The mean number of community nurse days is highest in the later years (20 or more 1983–86), while social worker contacts tend to be fewer in these years, with no contacts at all recorded in 1986. Day-centre facilities were much more used than day hospitals, the latter being used by one patient only in most years.

Table 39 compares the use of National Health Service (NHS) and local authority services (non-residential) in terms of contact days. It is clear that the use of the local authority services was substantial and that the day-centre days alone were more than twice the total NHS days. From this it is evident that if the use of part-3 accommodation and local authority hostels was also taken into account, the discharge of even this relatively small number of patients has

TABLE 37

Number of patients [1] using each service by year

Service	1979	1980	1981	1982	1983	1984	1985	1986
Psychiatric in-patient department	2	1	2	2	5	4	2	2
Out-patient department	7	7	4	5	6	4	3	3
Community psychiatric nurse	7	7	9	8	4	5	4	3
Social worker	6	7	7	6	7	2	3	–
Day centre	5	6	5	6	6	5	5	4
Day hospital	1	1	1	1	2	1	1	1
Domiciliary visit from a psychiatrist	2	–	1	1	1	1	1	–

1. Patients may appear more than once in this table.

TABLE 38

Mean number of days per patient using each service

Service	1979	1980	1981	1982	1983	1984	1985	1986
Psychiatric in-patient department	84	91	102	154	98	90	159	158
Out-patient department	3	4	5	3	4	5	4	3
Community psychiatric nurse	9	7	11	13	24	20	27	23
Social worker	14	13	14	15	8	2	9	–
Day centre	58	108	103	69	54	44	51	49
Day hospital	69	90	63	45	40	48	45	18
Domiciliary visit from a psychiatrist	1	–	1	1	1	1	1	–

TABLE 39

Comparison of contact days with non-residential services (NHS and local authority)

	1979	1980	1981	1982	1983	1984	1985	1986	Total
NHS									
domiciliary visit	2	1	–	1	1	1	1	–	7
day hospital	69	90	63	45	80	48	45	18	458
out-patient appointment	21	29	21	17	22	21	13	10	154
community psychiatric nurse	62	48	103	107	96	101	107	68	692
total	154	169	187	170	199	171	166	96	1312
Local authority									
social worker	85	94	99	92	50	2	27	2	451
day centre	292	646	516	413	323	219	255	196	2856
total	377	740	615	505	373	220	282	198	3311

implications for the community-based services, particularly those funded by the local authority, which made a major contribution to the support of these former Powick residents.

It is not possible to demonstrate any relationship between diagnosis or length of stay in Powick and the amount of use made of community support services, but there is a slight trend towards older patients using them less; this seems to be related to the fact that they were not only elderly but, in the main, living in local authority homes.

Cost of care

The figures for the cost of care are only available as at November 1985 (Table 40). The estimate of cost of care for discharged patients is therefore calculated only to the end of 1985.

TABLE 40

Patients discharged from Powick Hospital 31 December 1978 to 31 December 1985

No.	Months out of hospital	Individual service cost (£)							Total service cost (£)	Accommodation costs after discharge (£)	Mean cost per month (£)	Total cost (£)	Comparative Powick cost (£)
		d.t.	i.p.	o.p.	c.p.n.	d.h.	d.c.	s.w.					
1	68	–	1890	285	520	–	–	1080	3775	9044[1]	189	12 819	54 400
2	7	29	7182	–	13	–	–	–	7224	931	1165	8155	5600
3	36	–	–	–	–	–	–	–	–	18 000	500	18 000	28 800
4	46	–	13 284	–	–	–	–	–	13 284	23 000	789	36 284	36 800
5	81	58	10 476	75	247	–	2550	288	13 694	30 224[1]	542	43 918	64 800
6	47	–	–	15	260	–	–	2136	2411	20 210	481	22 621	37 600
7	81	–	–	15	–	8910	–	–	8925	40 500	610	49 425	64 800
8	80	–	–	30	–	–	15 198	1152	16 380	23 659[1]	500	40 039	64 000
9	80	–	270	525	351	–	7531	1176	9853	14 798[1]	308	24 651	64 000
10	80	–	1188	480	1105	–	9163	1440	13 376	19 569[1]	412	32 945	64 000
11	79	58	43 902	510	2185	–	6256	1200	54 111	18 823[1]	923	72 934	63 200
12	11	–	–	–	–	–	–	–	–	5500	500	5500	8800
13	72	–	–	–	–	–	–	48	48	36 000	501	36 048	57 600
14	61	–	–	–	–	–	–	48	48	30 500	501	30 548	48 800
15	63	–	–	15	507	–	782	720	2024	22 692[1]	392	24 716	50 400
16	63	29	1998	195	2327	–	2295	1200	8044	8379[1]	261	16 423	50 400
17	7	–	–	–	52	–	–	–	52	3500	507	3552	5600
18	41	29	–	–	–	–	–	–	29	20 500	501	20 529	32 800
19	39	29	25 002	15	–	770	–	120	25 936	19 500	1165	35 436	31 200
20	33	–	–	–	–	–	–	120	120	19 200	585	19 320	26 400
21	28	–	–	–	–	–	1462	–	1462	14 000	552	15 462	22 400
22	13	–	–	–	416	–	–	144	560	4105[1]	359	4665	10 400
23	6	–	–	–	–	–	–	–	–	3000	500	3000	4800
24	2	–	–	–	–	–	–	–	–	1000	500	1000	1600
Total	232	232	105 192	2160	7983	9680	45 237	10 872	181 356	406 634	523	587 990	899 200

1. Includes social security benefit net of 'pocket money'
d.v., domiciliary visit; i.p., in-patient; o.p., out-patient; c.p.n., community psychiatric nurse; d.h., day hospital; d.c., day centre; s.w., social worker.

It is possible to form an estimate of the costs of the pattern of care received by the 24 patients who were discharged from hospital (up to the end of 1985) and remained in the Worcester Project Area, by applying the costing techniques described in the Worcester Development Project Costing Manual (Stilwell, 1981, unpublished) and by making an estimate of social security entitlement. The single person's pension in November 1985 was £38.30. Of this, £7.65 would be payable as pocket money to patients in hospital, so a figure of £30.65 was used as an estimate of extra social security payments made to patients in the community, rather than hospital care.

This estimate is only approximate since other allowances are made in certain circumstances, and in some cases a family's entitlement is reduced by less than this amount when one member goes to hospital.

The average cost per month after discharge (November 1985 prices) was £523, compared with £800 which would have been the approximate in-patient cost at Powick or a similar mental hospital, disallowing the run down of Powick before closure. The largest element of the cost was that of accommodation/social security payments, being some 70% of the total. Only five patients cost less than half their hypothetical in-patient costs, and three actually cost more, mainly because of the length of time they subsequently spent as in-patients in the much more expensive Newtown Hospital. Another patient cost only 1.5% less than if he had remained at Powick, again because of treatment as an in-patient at Newtown.

There is a continuing debate about the relative costs of community versus hospital care, although the choice of community or in-patient care for a patient does not normally hinge on cost considerations. The experience of these 24 patients confirms that for the most part community care is cheaper by some 30–40%, but the cost of this type of care, as opposed to long-term in-patient care, can still be substantial if (even short-term) admission to a new psychiatric unit is required.

Discussion

It has become clear that closing a traditional mental hospital with its nucleus of aging long-term patients is not easy. In the first two years after admissions ceased, 20 patients were discharged (as opposed to transferred to another hospital); the following six years saw only ten discharges. Furthermore it was only in the years 1979 and 1980 that patients were discharged into the community or to sheltered accommodation – the later discharges were all to part-3 accommodation or a nursing home, with one patient going to a hostel.

Patients who were discharged made substantial demands on the community services (in particular social services) and part-3 accommodation. The experience of the Powick patients is similar to that reported by workers at Mapperley Hospital, Nottingham (Howat & Kontny, 1982). They found some of their discharged (long-term) patients were readmitted, but that none remained for extended periods; they also noted a high degree of dependence on day-care facilities. Significantly they report that "there was little evidence of further movement by the patients towards independence". Certainly only two of the Powick discharges moved to less sheltered accommodation than that to which they had been discharged. Others moved towards more sheltered living rather than less. It should be remembered, however, that apart from their mental illness, these patients were also elderly and that admission to part-3 accommodation, or more latterly a nursing home, might have been necessary if they had been living in the community all their lives.

The resident population still in hospital poses a tremendous problem. Since Tooth & Brooke (1961) published their study of the run down of the mental hospital population, there have been other attempts to forecast the run down of individual hospitals. In the mid-1960s the long-stay (two years or more) population was assessed at Powick (Cross *et al*, 1970), and it was estimated that 46% of the 1960 long-stay patients would still be in residence at the end of ten years. In the event, the proportion remaining was 42%, a difference of 33 patients. In 1979, this time with the aid of the psychiatric case register, a further study (Hassall & Cross, 1979) was made using three different methods. From these three methods it was estimated that of the 343 persons in residence when the hospital was closed to admissions, there would be between 220 and 240 remaining at the end of two years – there were 234: for 1982 the prediction was between 175 and 189 – there were 198; the forecast for the end of 1986 was 113 residents – one fewer than was actually the case. Making this type of prediction is not easy, and the further away from the date of the exercise, the more likely it is that the estimate will deviate from the true population.

It is important to try to make forecasts so that the problem of the remaining hospital residents can be realistically addressed. The economic consequences of maintaining a traditional mental hospital (with all that implies in terms of buildings), housing only a fraction of the number of patients for which it was built, have been discussed by Gillard (1984), but, in précis, although the bed occupancy fell by 51% from 1977–78 to 1981–82, expenditure fell by only 41%, and this trend continues. It is a matter of some urgency therefore to acquire suitable accommodation outside the hospital.

In 1985 a new survey of the in-patients was made, this time with the emphasis on finding out the needs of individual patients rather than trying to fit them into the existing pattern of care. From this survey it was clear that a range of facilities would be needed, from a few places for self-care to rather more places for high-supervision patients. At present just over a third of the population is under 65 (41 patients), which makes the time that these patients are likely to need accommodation outside hospital substantial, especially if they emulate the 11 residents currently aged 90 years or more.

The idea has been advanced that patients who came from outside the catchment area should be returned to their original area: in common with other mental hospitals, Powick has a sizeable proportion of such patients. There are several arguments against this – it would be a considerable upheaval for patients who may well have been at the host hospital for 20 years or more; in most cases all links have been lost with the place that they came from. Experience has shown that the areas from which these patients were originally transferred are unwilling to accept them. If they can stay in the Worcester area it is true that they will still have to face a move to unfamiliar surroundings, but at least they will be with fellow patients and staff that they know in a geographically familiar area.

Closure of a large mental hospital is a complex procedure. In many ways Powick was thought to be ideal for the experiment. The expansion of community services under the Development Project promised well for the patients to be discharged, and in the event would appear to give sufficient support to allow long-term patients to live, for the most part, outside the hospital, albeit in sheltered accommodation. Since a vigorous discharge policy has been pursued, it is reasonable to suppose that the remaining patients are unsuitable for existing facilities. Thus the need for specialist provision must be addressed if the hospital is to close.

A case register has been used in this study both to predict future trends in the hospital population and to monitor the use of the psychiatric services by the discharged patients. Because the case register is designed to record the psychiatric services, patients who were in part-3 or sheltered accommodation and, latterly, private nursing homes, had to be traced by contacting these agencies. We did not explore the question of how those who were discharged felt about leaving the hospital and their life outside it; this is an important dimension, but outside the remit of the present study.

The Worcester Development Project was designed to close the traditional mental hospital, replacing it with general hospital psychiatric units and extended, community-based services. The psychiatric units are open and working well, and the area has a well integrated network of community services, but the hospital has not closed. However, some valuable lessons have been learned about the strategy involved in such an exercise.

Summary

As a first step towards the closure of Powick Hospital the community-based services in the catchment area were improved and extended. In 1978 two new in-patient units were opened and a substantial number of patients from Powick were transferred to these facilities: at the end of the year Powick was closed to admissions. Long-term patients discharged since this time have made substantial demands on health and social services (particularly the latter), but none have returned to 'chronic' in-patient care.

At the end of 1986, 114 patients remained in Powick, most of whom are unlikely to be suitable for any of the residential accommodation that is currently available, even if there were sufficient places. It has become clear that although the enhancement of community resources and provision of new in-patient units are essential precursors to the closure of a mental hospital, more are needed if the hospital is to close within a decade of the cessation of admissions. Specialist residential accommodation will have to be provided outside the hospital for the remaining in-patients. Realistic provision demands that attempts be made to forecast the 'lifetime' of this population, since most of these patients will need specialist care for the rest of their lives.

Acknowledgement

We are indebted to Mr J. A. Stilwell, Senior Lecturer CRIBA, Warwick University, for the section on costs of care.

References

CROSS, D. W., HASSALL, C. & SPENCER, A. M. (1970) The dynamics of a long-stay mental hospital population. *British Journal of Preventive and Social Medicine*, **24**, 177–181.

DEPARTMENT OF HEALTH AND SOCIAL SECURITY (1970) *Feasibility Study for a Model Reorganisation of Mental Illness Services*. London: HMSO.

GILLARD, R. (1984) Keeping chins up as services run down. *Health and Social Services Journal*, 5 April.

HASSALL, C. (1976) The Worcester Development Project. *International Journal of Health*, **5**, 44–50.

—— & CROSS, K. W. (1979) Closing a mental hospital to admissions: predictions and predicaments. *Hospital and Health Services Review*, November, 393–395.

HOWAT, J. G. M. & KONTNY, E. L. (1982) The outcome for discharged Nottingham long-stay in-patients. *British Journal of Psychiatry*, **141**, 590–594.

MARKWICK, M. (1980) Breaking away from the routine. *Social Work Today*, **11**, 12–13.

TOOTH, G. C. & BROOKE, E. (1961) Trends in the mental hospital population and their effect on future planning. *Lancet*, i, 710.

III. Comparative studies

6 Community psychiatric nursing services in Salford, Southampton and Worcester

K. WOOFF, S. ROSE and J. STREET

The House of Commons Social Services Committee (1985) described the community psychiatric nurse (CPN) as a "key part of the new mental illness service" and quoted the Director of the Hospital Advisory Service, who wrote, "the CPN is probably the most important single professional in the process of moving care of mental illness into the community".

Although precise figures are not available, there is no doubt that CPN services have expanded rapidly during recent years. In 1978 the Community Psychiatric Nurses' Association estimated that there were 1500 staff of charge nurse grade and above engaged in community work; by 1984 its estimate was 3500 (see the Association's evidence to the House of Commons Social Services Committee (1985), Q1829).

The general enthusiasm for CPN services has not so far been informed by epidemiological data. Much early literature, reviewed by Griffith & Mangen (1980), concentrated on the discussion of various role definitions and unsystematic descriptions of individual services. Systematic studies, for example by Hunter (1978), Sladden (1979), and Paykel et al (1982), have described the activities of CPNs over a relatively short period of time. Apart from case register data from Salford (Wooff et al, 1986), we have been unable to find published data that compare services in different areas or show how CPN services have evolved over time.

The aim here is to describe, in epidemiological terms, the CPN services in three register areas, and their evolution over time.

The organisation of CPN services, and data collection methods

Salford

The CPN service began in 1973 with three full-time nurses. It was consultant based, and its purpose was to follow up patients who failed to attend for out-patient consultations or for phenothiazine injections. In January 1979, as a result of an experimental attachment of two nurses to general practices for three months, all CPNs moved from a hospital/consultant base to primary care community bases and began to accept referrals directly from general practitioners (GPs) and other primary health care staff. In 1984, only 16% of patients referred for CPN care were referred by psychiatrists.

Up to the end of 1983, all CPNs offered a generic service. Since then, some CPNs have been attached to psychogeriatric, drug, and alcohol specialist teams. The numbers of CPNs employed in the generic service expanded steadily, and by October 1982 18 nurses were in post.

Referral and discharge dates are extracted by a register clerk from the routine records kept centrally by the CPN department. Regular visits to the health centre bases are made to obtain more detailed data, to check queries and to collect information concerning phenothiazine injections. All cases, whether seen by psychiatrists or not, are recorded in the data bank. Where there has been no contact with a psychiatrist, the clinical category coded is that assigned by the CPN. In all other cases, the clinical category assigned by a psychiatrist is recorded.

Southampton

The CPN service began in 1968. Since 1973 it has been divided into two parts: a 'psychogeriatric' service for patients aged 65 and over, and an 'adult' service for patients aged between 15 and 64. Each service has its own nursing officer. The adult service also encompasses a specialist rehabilitation team. These services cover catchment areas that extend beyond the boundaries of the City of Southampton, and staffing figures have been adjusted accordingly.

Both adult and psychogeriatric services are hospital based, and operate an 'open' referral system. In practice, approximately 80% of referrals come from psychiatrists; the remainder come directly from patients themselves, or from GPs.

For the period covered by this study, people referred to CPN services who had never been seen by a psychiatrist, either before or after the referral date, were not included in the register data bank. This could involve a maximum of 20% of all referrals, but it is considered likely that the majority of these patients would have been found to have had contact with a psychiatrist at some time before or after their CPN referral.

Information about each patient receiving CPN care is collected quarterly, from each nurse, by register staff. Referral and discharge dates are recorded. There was some under-recording of referrals before 1980, and data before then should be interpreted with caution.

Worcester

A hospital-based CPN service started in Worcester at Powick Hospital in 1969. Referrals from all consultants were shared by the CPN team. Following the closure of Powick Hospital in 1978, two new psychiatric units opened in Worcester and Kidderminster, and a CPN team was attached to each unit.

In Worcester, CPNs were attached to each consultant, who was in turn responsible for psychiatric care in a particular geographical area; CPNs did not accept 'open' referrals until 1985. CPNs had mixed case loads until 1983, when a consultant-based psychogeriatric CPN team was set up.

In Kidderminster, a generic, hospital-based CPN service operated until the end of 1980, when a team of CPNs working with psychogeriatric patients only was established. An 'open' referral system has been in operation since 1978, but until 1982, when, following a 'publicity drive' direct GP referrals increased, only a very small proportion of referrals came direct from GPs. A 'diagnosis' of 'not known' was allotted to those patients referred by GPs who did not have contact with a psychiatrist, but following a recent increase in direct referrals from GPs, broad clinical categories assigned by the nurses with the assistance of a consultant psychiatrist when necessary, will be recorded on the register.

Definitions

Psychiatric patients have a mixture of chronic, acute and intermittent mental health problems, but there are no generally agreed definitions of 'chronic', 'acute' or 'intermittent' in service terms. In the absence of data on the natural history of many psychiatric disorders, period prevalence rates have been used to describe service utilisation over time.

Year prevalence, i.e. numbers or rates of patients seen in one year, has two components: the point or one-day prevalence at the start of each year, and 'new episodes', i.e. all patients seen during each year who did not appear in the preceding point-prevalence count. Some of the latter will have been referred for CPN care for the first time ever (inceptors), and some will have been re-referred after a break in care.

Year prevalence 1976–83

The large variations in total year prevalence illustrated in Fig. 10 show that rates were not solely dependent upon staffing levels. In 1983 the mean year prevalence rate per nurse was 110.3 in Salford; 42.6 in Southampton and 53.7 in Worcester. At just under 30%, proportions of inceptors to total year prevalence in 1982 and 1983 in Southampton were the lowest, with Salford and Worcester much the same at around 40%. The high Salford year prevalence rates cannot therefore solely be accounted for by high proportions of first-ever contacts.

Because data on CPN patients who have never seen a psychiatrist are excluded from the Southampton data bank, interpretation of area differences in the proportion of CPN patients who were not in touch with psychiatrists must be speculative. Figures that are available show that in 1983, in Salford 72% of patients in the CPN point-prevalence count had not seen any other member of the psychiatric team for at least 90 days; the equivalent proportion in Southampton was 25%. Proportions were rising in Salford, and falling in Southampton. Point prevalence data are not available from Worcester.

Additional staff time may be used in a variety of ways. Existing patients may receive more intensive care, there may be a build up of 'old' patients who continue to be cared for as before, or the services may take on more 'new' patients.

In Salford the mean year prevalence rate per nurse rose from 78.4 in 1976 to 126.3 in 1980; it then declined each year and in 1983 was 110.3. In Southampton, although rates were lower, they moved in the same direction as Salford's, with rises from 33.4 in 1978 to 67.5 in 1981, followed by falls in each subsequent year to 42.6 in 1983. In Worcester, mean year prevalence rates

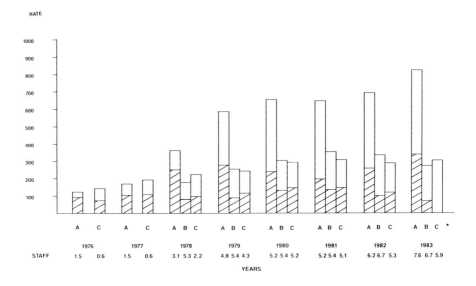

RATE

STAFF

YEARS

Fig. 10. Community psychiatric nursing services, year prevalences 1976–83 and first-ever CPN contact ▨ . Rates per 100 000 total population, (A) Salford, (B) Southampton and (C) Worcester. Staff = WTE per 100 000 total population as at 1 July each year. *Unavailable

per nurse fell dramatically from 234.5 in 1976 to 56.1 in 1979 and remained steady thereafter.

The proportions of 'old' and 'new' cases varied over time. In Salford, the proportions of 'new' cases fell from 73% in 1976 to 31% in 1981 and rose to 39% in 1982 and 42% in 1983. The proportions of inceptions in Southampton fell from 41% in 1978 to 26% in 1983. There was no clear trend in Worcester, where proportions remained around 47% between 1976 and 1980, but fell to 41% by 1983.

Clinical category and age

The clinical groupings (see footnote to Table 5 for definitions) of CPN cases in the various areas are shown in Table 41. In 1982, similar proportions (around 30%) of patients with schizophrenia or paranoid psychoses were seen in all three districts. Compared to those in Southampton and Worcester, Salford CPNs had very low proportions of patients in the 'affective psychoses' group (7% compared to 17% and 16% respectively). However, they had high proportions of 'other depressions' (29% compared to 11% and 12%); 'other neuroses' (13% compared to 3% and 6%); and 'personality disorders' (9% compared to 4% and 5%). Proportions in the 'dementia' group were over twice as high in Southampton as in Salford and Worcester.

In 1982 rates increased with age in all areas. In Southampton, this increase was particularly steep, with patients aged 75 and over forming 32% of the total

TABLE 41

CPN services: year prevalence rates per 100 000 total population 1976, 1978, 1980 and 1982 by clinical group

Clinical group	Area	1976	1978	1980	1982
Schizophrenia/paranoid psychoses	Salford	50.8	147.2	209.3	185.2
	Southampton		72.0	102.3	115.0
	Worcester	62.4	77.7	88.8	91.5
Affective psychosis	Salford	10.3	35.5	52.9	48.7
	Southampton		41.0	64.0	57.7
	Worcester	20.9	35.6	47.3	47.8
Other depression	Salford	22.5	71.8	171.3	203.9
	Southampton		27.1	45.6	38.6
	Worcester	15.8	24.3	37.5	36.0
Alcohol/drug disorders	Salford	3.0	9.9	20.6	25.4
	Southampton		1.9	5.3	2.9
	Worcester	5.7	7.8	29.5	14.5
Other neuroses	Salford	11.8	34.7	81.2	89.9
	Southampton		10.5	13.6	10.8
	Worcester	13.9	14.7	21.5	19.4
Dementia	Salford	3.8	16.8	43.6	43.7
	Southampton		8.1	42.2	77.8
	Worcester	8.2	18.1	30.1	30.0
Other organic	Salford	1.5	3.8	7.7	8.7
	Southampton		5.7	14.1	11.7
	Worcester	2.2	2.5	5.2	6.7
Personality disorders	Salford	7.6	19.1	42.8	62.0
	Southampton		6.6	11.6	14.2
	Worcester	6.7	11.9	14.1	13.6
All other	Salford	6.1	21.4	27.1	36.6
	Southampton		3.3	6.3	14.0
	Worcester	4.8	12.8	25.2	40.0
Total	Salford	117.6	356.3	656.6	704.2
	Southampton	175.5	304.9	342.5	
	Worcester	140.7	205.3	299.1	299.5

year prevalence. Other characteristics of the psychogeriatric service in Southampton are described in Chapter 2. Proportions in Salford and Worcester were similar, with patients in the 25–44 and 45–64 age ranges forming around 30% each of the total year prevalence. Patients in the oldest age group formed 13% and 17% of the total respectively.

The breakdowns of clinical categories within each age group (see also Table 42) varied between register areas. In 1982 in the 25–44 and 45–64 age groups, patients in the schizophrenia and paranoid psychoses group were the most numerous in all areas, but proportions varied between 27% and 33% respectively in Salford, 35% and 43% in Worcester, and 54% and 50% in Southampton. Salford had the highest proportions of patients in the 'other depression' clinical group (29%) – in Worcester equivalent proportions were 12% and 11%, and in Southampton they were 5% and 9%. In the oldest age group the main clinical category was dementia, but again proportions varied between 30% in Salford, 41% in Worcester and 50% in Southampton. Salford and Southampton had the same proportions of schizophrenia and paranoid psychoses (14%); the proportion in Worcester was 8%. 'Other depressions' were 12% in Worcester, 13% in Southampton, and 26% in Salford.

Proportions of patients in the schizophrenia and paranoid psychoses group declined by about 10% over time everywhere. In Salford, changes in the

TABLE 42
CPN services: year prevalence rates per 100 000 population aged 15 and over 1976, 1978, 1980 and 1982, by age group

Age group	Area	1976	1978	1980	1982
15–24	Salford	63.0	133.6	311.7	351.5
	Southampton		33.7	62.2	51.2
	Worcester	50.7	56.4	108.9	109.4
25–44	Salford	187.2	532.3	909.7	936.0
	Southampton		182.3	265.8	249.9
	Worcester	197.0	248.4	341.5	311.2
45–64	Salford	161.5	532.9	927.5	964.8
	Southampton		321.9	384.0	387.0
	Worcester	223.9	317.6	446.7	423.4
65–74	Salford	200.3	577.1	1053.5	1036.1
	Southampton		342.0	744.1	786.7
	Worcester	213.0	401.5	561.2	557.0
75 and over	Salford	131.5	707.6	1156.1	1490.4
	Southampton		410.6	1265.0	1818.6
	Worcester	225.1	409.1	700.5	901.6
Total (15 and over)	Salford	152.2	468.7	829.5	877.2
	Southampton		223.9	381.8	425.0
	Worcester	181.5	262.5	379.3	378.1

diagnostic composition of CPN patients were emphasised when the service shifted from a hospital to a community base. The relatively high proportions of patients in the dementia category in Southampton were probably due to the establishment of a specialist psychogeriatric team. The increase in the proportion of patients in the 'other' category in 1982 in Worcester was likely to have been the result of an expansion of referrals from GPs, and further details of the precise nature of this expansion will be possible when more data on the clinical categories of such patients become available. Proportions in other clinical categories in Southampton and Worcester changed little over time.

Proportions in the youngest age group remained steady over time in all three areas. Proportions in the 24–44 and 45–64 age ranges fell slightly in Salford and Worcester, and more dramatically in Southampton, where a decline of 40% between 1978 and 1982 affected proportionately more patients aged between 45 and 64 in the affective psychosis category.

In Southampton, proportions in the 65–74 age group rose slowly from 17% in 1978 to 21% in 1982; the high rate of expansion in the over 75 group (from 13% to 32% between 1978 and 1982) occurred mainly in the dementia category. Proportions of elderly patients in the schizophrenia and paranoid psychoses group remained steady.

Other hospital services

Data in this section are taken from Gibbons *et al* (1984). After 1976 in-patient admission rates in the 15–64 age group rose in Southampton and Worcester and tended to decline slightly in Salford. In Salford and Worcester, the proportions of these patients in the schizophrenia and paranoid psychoses category were stable; in Southampton they rose by approximately 10%.

Proportions of admissions in the 'other depressions' group stayed the same in Salford, and fell in Southampton and Worcester. In the over 65 age range, admissions increased in all areas. As a result of operating a relief admission service, admission rates in Southampton rose considerably.

In Worcester between 1976 and 1983, there was a 50% and 25% reduction in the proportions of patients in the 15–64 and over 65 age groups who had been continuously in hospital between one and five years. In Salford, equivalent proportions increased by 37% and 83% respectively; in Southampton there was an increase of 8% in the 15–64 age range and a reduction of 5% in those over 65.

In Salford and Worcester, rates for people aged between 15 and 64 attending psychiatric out-patient clinics rose by 10% and 20% respectively between 1976 and 1981. In Southampton, rates declined by 14%. In all three areas rates of people aged over 65 attending for out-patient care rose substantially.

Discussion

Although all three services evolved differently, they shared two important characteristics. Overall staffing levels were very similar, and they all, in spite of some variation, accumulated a substantial proportion of 'chronic' patients. In Salford and Worcester, the proportions of 'first-ever' CPN contacts per nurse levelled out in recent years; in Southampton proportions continued to fall.

The Salford service, based on attachment to GPs, was characterised by larger case loads, little involvement with patients in the affective psychoses group, but high involvement with patients in the 'other depression' and 'anxiety' categories, and large numbers of patients who received care from CPNs only. Although the numbers of psychotic patients cared for by the CPNs rose over time, the vast majority of 'new' referrals came directly via GPs and were primarily of non-psychotic patients. Other data show that mean time in therapeutic contact with psychotic patients was considerably lower (nine minutes) than with neurotic patients (25 minutes) and was almost entirely devoted to the administration of an injection. Thus a change away from caring for psychotic patients has already begun and contacts with other specialist mental health staff have been observed to be limited (Wooff *et al*, 1986, 1988). This situation is associated with the accumulation of 'new' long-stay in-patients at a similar rate to that pertaining in the late 1960s.

In Southampton, services for the elderly expanded considerably. Case loads were the lowest of all three areas, and the accumulation of 'chronic' patients the highest. The bulk of the elderly patients were in the dementia group. This service, together with the use of short term relief in-patient beds, apparently succeeded in reducing the rate at which elderly 'new' long-stay in-patients accumulated.

In Worcester, sizes of case loads and 'turnover' were higher than in Southampton, but considerably lower than in Salford. The client 'mix' remained much the same throughout the period although, in common with other areas, the proportion of patients in the schizophrenia and paranoid psychoses group declined somewhat. There was a substantial reduction in the accumulation of 'new' long-stay in-patients of all ages.

The style of the Salford service clearly varied considerably from that in Southampton and Worcester. Although differences in size of case load may to some extent be accounted for by the urban/rural factor, it is unlikely that the large case loads carried in Salford and the very short contact times with psychotic patients offer much opportunity for intensive therapeutic intervention. Very few (16% in 1984) referrals came from psychiatrists, and it was observed that the CPNs in Salford were devoting the bulk of their time to working with patients who were unlikely to be 'at risk' of becoming long-term in-patients. The other two CPN services, both hospital based, were associated with decreasing reliance on long-term in-patient care.

It is often the case that care staff respond to the immediate demands made upon them, irrespective of whether those 'demands' coincide with overall 'need' or with service objectives. The data presented here indicate how CPN services, variously organised in ways that expose staff to different kinds of demands, may evolve. Members of the House of Commons Select Committee on Social Services (1985) expressed their concern that CPNs may be "tempted away from a specialist role towards becoming additional district nurses or social workers". The data presented here suggest that the acceptance of direct referrals from GPs, and attachment to primary care teams, may lead to the very situation the Select Committee feared. They also show that staff increases alone will not automatically result in increases in individual client contact times and that they may equally well result in the same kind of service being given to more clients.

The CPN services are relatively new, and planners and managers whose previous management experience is likely to have been within the confines of institutions must recognise the difficulties of ensuring that scarce specialist psychiatric nursing resources are used where they are most appropriate. Unless role boundaries are clearly defined, training in specific therapeutic techniques given, and 'clinical supervision' of case loads instituted, psychotic clients and their families may not benefit from any increase in CPN resources. The implications for increased training resources, not least for the CPN managers, are clear.

References

GIBBONS, J., JENNINGS, C. & WING, J. K. (1984) *Psychiatric Care in Eight Register Areas*. Southampton: University Department of Psychiatry. (Copies obtainable by sending £2.50, cheque payable to University of Southampton, to University Department of Psychiatry, Royal South Hants Hospital, Southampton SO9 4PE.)

GRIFFITH, J. H. & MANGEN, S. P. (1980) Community psychiatric nursing – a literature review. *International Journal of Nursing Studies*, **17**, 197–210.

HOUSE OF COMMONS SOCIAL SERVICES COMMITTEE (1985) *Second Report, Community Care with Special Reference to Adult Mentally Ill and Mentally Handicapped People, 1984–85* (HC13-I). London: HMSO.

HUNTER, P. (1978) *Schizophrenia and Community Psychiatric Nursing*. London: National Schizophrenia Fellowship.

PAYKEL, E. S., MANGEN, S. P., GRIFFITH, J. H., *et al* (1982) Psychiatric nursing for neurotic patients: a controlled trial. *British Journal of Psychiatry*, **140**, 573–581.

SLADDEN, S. (1979) *Psychiatric Nursing in the Community. A Study of the Working Situation*. University of Edinburgh, Department of Nursing, Monograph No. 6. Edinburgh: Churchill Livingstone.

WOOFF, K., GOLDBERG, D. P. & FRYERS, T. (1986) Patients in receipt of community psychiatric nursing care in Salford 1976–82. *Psychological Medicine*, **16**, 407–414.

——, —— & —— (1988) The practice of community psychiatric nursing and mental health social work in Salford. Some implications for community care. *British Journal of Psychiatry*, **152**, 783–792.

7 The use of psychiatric services by the elderly: a study based on the case registers of Nottingham, Salford, Southampton and Worcester

**S. JONES, C. HASSALL, C. JENNINGS
and M. CLEVERLY**

In recent years there has been an increase in the size of the elderly population of the UK, but this has not been spread evenly across age bands. For instance, between 1971 and 1981, the total population of England rose by only 0.5%, but those aged 65–74 years increased by 7%, those aged 75–84 years by 20%, and those over 85 years by 19%. Increases of this magnitude affect the demand for psychiatric services, since the elderly have been shown to make greater use of them. This was evident in the first inter-register report (Gibbons *et al*, 1984), in which tables were presented that followed the convention of grouping all the elderly persons over 65 years old into one large category. This convention is followed almost universally in local, regional and national service statistics, but in view of the differentials noted above, a more detailed examination of service use by the elderly is essential.

Four of the UK psychiatric case registers therefore decided to collaborate in a preliminary study of psychiatric service use by the elderly. The data presented in this chapter complement those in Chapter 2. Two groups of patients were selected: (a) new referrals to the service and (b) resident in-patients. Two index years, several years apart, were studied for each of these groups, to examine for consistency between the case registers and to detect any obvious trends over time.

New referrals were examined in terms of their mode of entry to the services and the care they received in the three months following first contact: the two years chosen were 1978 and 1982. Resident in-patients were described in terms of their use of psychiatric services during the two years before and after the censal dates (31 December 1976 and 31 December 1981). Both new and resident patients were examined in four age groups: 15–64, 65–74, 75–84, and over 85 years. This involved small numbers in some of the older groups, with consequent difficulties in interpreting some results.

Three broad diagnostic categories were used (see footnote to Table 5 for definitions): (a) all types of depression and affective disorder (groups 2 and 3),

(b) all types of organic disorders (groups 6 and 7), and (c) all other diagnoses (groups 1, 4, 5, 8, and 9). Patients were defined as those people who had had a face-to-face contact with a psychiatrist; thus people who, for example, received psychiatric services only from psychiatric community nurses or social workers would not be defined as in psychiatric care.

New referrals to psychiatrists

Definitions

New patients in this study were defined as those having had no previous contact with a psychiatrist for two years or more. Patients were grouped according to their type of first contact with psychiatric services. The groupings used were:

(a) admission
(b) day care
(c) domiciliary visit
(d) contact following an episode of deliberate self-harm
(e) referrals from general hospital departments
(f) any other out-patient care

Type of follow-up contact within three months of first contact was grouped in the same way.

'Any other out-patient care' was broadly equivalent to non-emergency referrals, most patients in this category being seen in scheduled out-patient clinics. In the past these contacts would all have taken place in hospital clinics, but now such patients are often seen in general practice surgeries and community bases. In addition, an increasing number of doctors are undertaking non-urgent home assessments. Unlike traditional domiciliary visits, which are carried out in response to referrals that have at least some degree of urgency, these are not usually emergencies, but a displacement from scheduled clinics on hospital premises, in the same way that patients might be seen in general practice surgeries. In Nottingham, such non-urgent visits are not included with domiciliary visits but with 'any other out-patient care'. In the other three areas 'domiciliary visit' includes all home contacts regardless of urgency or initiator. Furthermore, in Worcester, domiciliary visits and ward liaison referrals are not separated. These differences in the definition of a domiciliary visit need to be borne in mind when comparing the extent and urgency of domiciliary care in each area.

Day care in this study was limited to that provided by the National Health Service (NHS). This meant that it predominantly reflects the use of acute day hospitals rather than day centres, and is less heterogeneous than if all forms of day care were included.

Total numbers of new patients referred to psychiatric services

The total number of patients referred increased slightly between 1978 and 1982 in Nottingham and Worcester but fell in Southampton and Salford. Table 43 shows

TABLE 43
New patients – total numbers of patients entering psychiatric care in 1978 and 1982 by age group

Age group	Nottingham			Salford			Southampton			Worcester		
	1978	1982	% change	1978	1982	% change	1978	1982	% change	1978	1982	% change
15–64	1783	1837	+ 3	1544	855	– 45	1126	928	– 18	892	897	+ 1
65–74	208	244	+ 17	212	178	– 16	142	164	+ 15	100	109	+ 9
75–84	228	287	+ 26	117	243	+ 108	168	230	+ 37	92	121	+ 32
85 and over	88	107	+ 22	25	66	+ 164	89	90	+ 1	26	39	+ 50
Total 65 and over	524	638	+ 22	354	487	+ 38	399	484	+ 21	218	269	+ 23
Total	2307	2475	+ 7	1898	1342	– 29	1525	1412	– 7	1110	1166	+ 5

that there were considerable differences between the two years for the individual age groups. The number of referred patients aged 15–64 rose slightly in Nottingham and Worcester, but fell in Southampton and Salford. The numbers of patients aged 65–74 rose in Nottingham, Southampton and Worcester, but declined in Salford. All areas experienced an increase in numbers of patients aged 75–84. In Nottingham, Southampton and Worcester this increase was around 30%, but there was a doubling of patient numbers in Salford in this age group. The number of patients aged over 85 showed no change in Southampton, increased by a fifth in Nottingham, by half in Worcester, and more than doubled in Salford.

In all four areas the sex and diagnostic distribution of patients was similar in both years, numerical changes merely reflecting the changes in total patient numbers. Overall the male:female ratio was 1:1.4. As might be expected, less than 5% of patients aged 15–64 had been given a diagnosis of organic psychosis, but 30% of those aged 65–74, 50% of those aged 74–85, and 70% of those aged over 85 fell into this diagnostic category. The proportion of patients with 'depression' diagnoses was between 40% and 50% in the age groups up to 84, but fell to include only 25% of those aged over 85. Around two-thirds of patients aged 15–64 were described as suffering from other psychiatric illness, but only 10–15% of those aged 65–84 and 5% of those aged over 85.

Type of first contact with psychiatric services

Although the likelihood of contact with psychiatric services is related to both sex and psychiatric diagnosis, the influence these variables have is probably fairly constant both between areas and over time. In contrast, the point of entry to psychiatric services is a function of both available facilities and local working practices, and as such showed considerable variation between the four areas. They are therefore discussed separately.

Nottingham

The overall pattern of type of first contact was similar in 1978 and 1982, the most significant difference between these years being the numbers of patients referred by general hospital doctors. Table 44 shows that there was a large increase in the number and proportion of patients referred from general hospital departments (not following an episode of deliberate self-harm). This dramatic

TABLE 44

New patients – percentage of each age group by type of first contact, 1978 and 1982

	Nottingham		Salford		Southampton		Worcester	
	1978	1982	1978	1982	1978	1982	1978	1982
Admission								
15–64	4	8	10	8	9	10	9	12
65–74	10	11	13	2	2	18	17	NK
75–84	7	6	23	2	4	2	22	18
85 and over	2	2	20	3	3	–	12	10
Day care								
15–64	0.2	0.5	1	0.7	2	3.5	0.1	1
65–74	0.5	1.6	1	0.6	1	0.6	–	1
75–84	4	0.7	–	–	0.6	–	3	1
85 and over	11	3	4	–	–	–	–	–
Domiciliary visit								
15–64	13	9	14	21	10	13	21	26
65–74	48	40	40	71	58	68	51	51
75–84	61	47	58	73	75	79	62	65
85 and over	57	40	68	82	76	74	88	82
Ward referral (excluding attempted suicide)								
15–64	4	7	1	1	12	4	NK	NK
65–74	5	17	2	12	17	14	NK	NK
75–84	7	19	2	12	17	21	NK	NK
85 and over	8	11	4	20	20	24	NK	NK
Attempted suicide								
15–64	25	21	1	NK	12	11	6	11
65–74	10	5	–	9	–	1	3	NK
75–84	4	3	2	NK	1	0.4	1	2
85 and over	1	2	–	NK	–	–	–	–
Other out-patient care								
15–64	53	55	72	NK	55	58	56	49
65–74	27	26	44	NK	13	5	30	28
75–84	18	25	15	NK	3	–	12	14
85 and over	20	42	4	NK	–	1	–	8

NK, not known.

increase reflects the introduction of a psychiatric liaison service in the two general hospitals in Nottingham between 1979 and 1980. In contrast, the number of patients seen following an episode of deliberate self-harm fell. This again is probably a reflection of the introduction of the liaison service, which is thought to have improved the assessment of patients by staff from the accident and emergency department. There has also been an increase in social work input in the screening of deliberate self-harm patients, further reducing the proportion actually seeing a psychiatrist.

The proportions of patients in each age group making their first contact in other forms of out-patient care were similar in both years. This largely represents patients seen in scheduled clinics and includes over 50% of patients aged 15–64. There was a shift of patients aged over 85 from domiciliary visits to other out-patient care. This may in fact be an artefact of recording methods, with scheduled home assessments being included in the other out-patient care category to a greater extent in 1982 than in 1978. Although home assessments were being undertaken in 1978 the number was minimal, and the need to differentiate between the two types of domiciliary visit was not always fully recognised. The decision by two clinical teams, in 1982, to undertake all first assessments at home whenever possible led to a clarification of definitions and the setting of rigorous guidelines.

Salford

The pattern of type of first contact for the 15–64 age group was similar in 1978 and 1982 with a slight increase in the proportion seen on domiciliary visits in 1982. The majority (70%) made their first contact in scheduled out-patient care. Patients in the age group 65–74 showed a decrease in admissions and an increase in ward referrals over time. First contacts in other forms of out-patient care fell and appeared to be replaced by domiciliary visits, which showed an increase. For patients aged 75–84, both domiciliary visits and ward referrals increased, while admission fell as a type of first contact. Domiciliary visits and ward referrals increased in the over 85 age group, with admissions showing a substantial decrease. Numbers of patients in this age group having day care, contact following an episode of deliberate self-harm, or other out-patient contact were negligible in each year. In all age groups there were very few contacts following deliberate self-harm in either year.

Southampton

The pattern of type of first contact for the 15–64 age group was similar in 1978 and 1982, with over 50% of patients having their first contact in other out-patient care. Admission was the point of first contact for 10% of patients. The proportion making contact with psychiatric services following a referral from a general hospital department (not associated with attempted suicide) fell from 12% in 1978 to only 4% in 1982.

The experience of patients in the age group 65–74 also showed little difference between the two years. The proportion having a domiciliary visit as their first contact rose between 1978 and 1982, while the proportion entering via other out-patient care fell. Southampton has a policy of domiciliary assessments for psychogeriatrics and the switch to domiciliary visits from other out-patient care may not reflect a rise in emergency visits, merely the replacement of assessment in out-patient clinics by home assessment.

The two age groups 75–84 and 85 and over entered services in much the same way in both 1978 and 1982. Around three-quarters of patients in these two age groups had their first contact as a domiciliary visit, again a reflection of the emphasis on home assessment of geriatric referrals.

Worcester

The pattern of type of first contact for all patients aged 15–64 was similar in both 1978 and 1982 with half being seen in routine out-patient care. There was an increase in the number seen following an episode of deliberate self-harm.

Patients in the older age groups also had a similar pattern of type of first contact in both years. Over half of those aged 65–74 were first seen on a domiciliary visit, 63% of those aged 75–84 and 85% of those aged over 85. There was a slight move from domiciliary visits to other out-patient contacts for patients aged 85 and over. However, domiciliary visits and ward referrals in Worcester are not differentiated, and it is thus not possible to determine whether one or both of these types of contact was decreasing.

Use of psychiatric services in the three months following first contact

The groupings of type of contact used for point of entry were also used to describe follow-up care in the three months following first contact. However, some events are more commonly associated with initial contact with psychiatric services. Referrals from general hospital departments (whether following a suicide attempt or not) accounted for 10–30% of first contacts, but are rare as follow-up events. By contrast, admission to in-patient or day patient care is likely to be more common as a follow-up event than initial entry to services, simply because it is commonly preceded by out-patient assessment of some kind. Subsequent care varied between areas, which are described separately.

Nottingham

Episodes of in-patient care fell for the two age groups comprising those patients aged 15–74, but remained stable for the older age groups. Table 45 shows that use of day care doubled for patients aged 15–64, but there was a tendency to declining use the older the patient age group. During the late 1970s and early '80s NHS day care in Nottingham was evolving from a mixture of day centres (which had been developed as part of the policy of discharging long-stay patients) and day hospitals, to being solely acute day hospitals. The marked drop in use of day care by the very old may to some extent be reflecting this change rather than a real reduction in the use of day hospitals. Other out-patient care (largely scheduled appointments) increased for all age groups.

TABLE 45

Use of psychiatric services in the three months after first contact – age-specific rates per 1000 population, 1978 and 1982

	No. of in-patient admissions		No. of episodes of day care		No. of domiciliary visits		No. of ward referrals (excluding attempted suicide)		No. of contacts through attempted suicide		No. of other out-patient contacts	
	1978	1982	1978	1982	1978	1982	1978	1982	1978	1982	1978	1982
Nottingham												
15–64	1.8	1.4	0.2	0.5	1.1	0.8	0.3	0.7	2.0	1.7	10.0	10.8
65–74	3.3	2.4	1.2	1.1	3.0	3.1	0.3	1.4	0.6	0.4	3.8	4.1
75–84	5.4	6.4	5.0	3.6	8.4	8.7	1.3	3.8	0.6	0.5	3.8	6.2
85 and over	8.1	9.4	11.0	3.0	14.2	12.6	1.9	4.0	0.3	0.5	7.2	13.4
Salford												
15–64	2.3	1.3	0.5	0.3	1.5	1.2	0.2	0.1	0.1	0.0	13.7	9.6
65–74	4.6	1.5	0.6	0.1	4.0	6.3	0.3	1.0	–	–	7.9	3.2
75–84	5.9	4.1	0.7	0.7	6.4	16.6	0.3	4.8	0.2	0.1	3.5	3.2
85 and over	8.1	6.0	1.0	–	8.1	28.1	0.5	7.8	–	–	1.0	0.5
Southampton												
15–64	2.0	2.1	0.8	0.5	1.8	1.6	1.2	0.5	1.1	0.9	12.7	11.2
65–74	4.0	2.8	0.7	0.4	16.6	29.1	2.3	2.8	0.8	–	2.7	1.6
75–84	8.9	9.8	0.5	0.6	40.2	64.5	6.4	6.8	0.2	0.1	1.0	0.2
85 and over	22.5	13.7	0.9	0.4	96.8	93.3	14.6	18.8	–	–	–	0.9
Worcester												
15–64	0.9	1.3	0.1	0.4	NK	NK	1.4	1.2	0.3	0.5	6.7	6.0
65–74	2.7	1.9	0.3	0.6	NK	NK	1.9	2.1	0.0	0.1	4.0	3.8
75–84	14.8	4.1	0.2	1.5	NK	NK	4.6	5.4	0.1	0.1	2.2	4.1
85 and over	3.0	5.0	0.9	0.6	NK	NK	7.1	10.7	–	–	3.6	2.1

NK, not known

Salford

Admissions decreased substantially for patients aged 65–74, and fell slightly for the other age groups. Use of day care increased for the 15–64 age group but declined for other age groups. Non-emergency and non-liaison contacts (other out-patient care) fell considerably for patients aged 15–74, remaining stable for the older patients.

Southampton

The use of in-patient care was similar in both years, while use of day care fell, mainly in the 15–64 age group. Domiciliary visits increased dramatically for the 65–84 age group, but remained the same for the very old and for those aged 15–64. The stability of the number of domiciliary visits for those over 85 may reflect the greater difficulty of maintaining people of this age in their own homes. The slight tendency for declining use of day care may be associated with the increased number of domiciliary visits, which might be viewed as an alternative means of maintaining people at home, which can be effected rather more quickly than decisions to increase the provision of day care. There are only minor changes in the other out-patient contacts.

Worcester

There were small changes in the number of admissions, except for the 75–84 age group, where there was a substantial decrease. All age groups showed a rise in episodes of day care, particularly 75–84, except for 85 and over, where there was a slight decrease.

Comparison between areas of type of first contact and subsequent care

Although facilities and working practices do vary between the four register areas, a surprising consistency was found in the use of services. As a crude indicator of the likelihood of any type of care being received, the numbers of episodes of in-patient and day care per patient were calculated in each of the four areas. Table 46 shows that, in general, patients aged 15–64 had fewer episodes of in-patient care than those aged over 65. All four areas showed similar patterns for episodes of in-patient care with a tendency for this to decline between 1978 and 1982. There was also a tendency for numbers of episodes per patient to be substantially higher the older the patient group. This difference was not as striking in 1982 as in 1978, possibly a reflection of the general decrease in the use of in-patient facilities.

The numbers of out-patient contacts, including domiciliary visits and general hospital referrals (following deliberate self-harm or not), were remarkably similar both between the two years and between areas. However, Southampton was slightly different from the other three areas in having a much higher rate per patient in both years, which undoubtedly reflects the domiciliary visiting policy in Southampton. The greater fall in the admission rate for those over 85 in Southampton, shown in Table 45, may be an indicator of the success of this policy. Salford and Southampton both showed an increase in the number

TABLE 46

New patients – spells of in-patient and day patient care and numbers of out-patient contacts per patient in first three months, 1978 and 1982

	Admissions per patient		Spells of day care per patient		Out-patient contacts per patient	
	1978	1982	1978	1982	1978	1982
Nottingham						
15–64	0.3	0.2	0.0	0.1	1.9	1.9
65–74	0.6	0.3	0.2	0.2	1.3	1.3
75–84	0.4	0.4	0.4	0.2	1.0	1.1
85 and over	0.3	0.3	0.5	0.1	1.0	1.1
Salford						
15–64	0.2	0.2	0.1	0.1	1.6	2.0
65–74	0.5	0.2	0.1	0.0	1.4	1.4
75–84	0.6	0.2	0.1	0.0	1.0	1.2
85 and over	0.7	0.2	0.1	0.0	0.8	1.2
Southampton						
15–64	0.2	0.3	0.1	0.1	2.0	2.3
65–74	0.5	0.3	0.1	0.0	2.9	3.7
75–84	0.5	0.4	0.0	0.0	2.7	3.2
85 and over	0.5	0.4	0.0	0.0	2.7	3.0
Worcester						
15–64	0.2	0.3	0.0	0.1	1.9	1.8
65–74	0.8	0.5	0.1	0.2	1.7	1.6
75–84	0.4	0.5	0.1	0.2	0.9	1.2
85 and over	0.4	0.4	0.1	0.1	1.5	1.1

of out-patient contacts per patient between the two years, while Nottingham and Worcester remained stable. The number of episodes of day care per patient was very small in all areas for all age groups and any differences between the years are thus difficult to interpret.

Differences in the pattern of care received by people referred to psychiatric services in the four areas were largely explicable in terms of the different service provision. For instance, the increase in patients seen following a referral from a general hospital doctor in Nottingham occurred after the introduction of a specific psychiatric liaison service in the general hospitals. Similarly, the increase in the number of domiciliary visits to those over 65 in Southampton followed the development of a psychogeriatric service. An age gradient was apparent. For instance, the majority (50–70%) of people aged 15–64 had their first contact in other out-patient care (scheduled clinics), with 10–20% seen on domiciliary visits (mostly emergencies). These proportions changed for each age group, so that the majority of the over 85 age group were being seen on domiciliary visits.

In general both type of first contact and follow-up care for patients aged 65–74 were more similar to the pattern for patients aged 15–64 than to the older age groups. However, the pattern of use of psychiatric services for patients aged over 75 was substantially different. When all patients aged over 65 are considered as a single group these differences become blurred simply because the total population aged 65–74 is almost double that aged over 75. This suggests that 65 may not be the most appropriate cut off in defining the elderly in service terms. The major changes in service use occurring after the age of 75 indicate that a subdivision of the elderly into at least 65–74 and over 75 is justified.

Resident in-patients

Definitions

Two censal dates were chosen, 31 December 1976 and 31 December 1981. All resident in-patients from the appropriate catchment area of each register were identified on each of these dates and divisions made by sex, diagnosis, and age, in the same way as for the new entrants to psychiatric services. Data were obtained on the care received by patients for both the two years before and the two years after each censal date. This included numbers of in-patient and day-patient episodes and out-patient contacts (of any type) in each two-year period. Once again, psychiatric care was defined as contact with a psychiatrist, and thus excluded contact that was maintained only with professionals such as social workers and community nurses.

Total numbers of resident patients

The diagnostic distribution for resident in-patients (Table 47) was broadly similar between the four areas. Diagnostic information is usually collected as part of routine clinical practice and thus may be obtained from a large number of doctors. Differences in diagnosis between areas may thus be partly a reflection of diagnostic habits rather than differences in patient groups.

Nottingham

A similar diagnostic distribution of resident in-patients was found in both years. The age distribution in both years was also similar, although there was an overall drop of 3% in the number of resident in-patients.

Salford

Although the total number of in-patients was similar for the two years in Salford there was an increase in the proportion of older patients. This was expected in view of the aging population of the area. The number of in-patients with a diagnosis of organic psychosis increased by 19% for males and by 59% for females over the five-year period, predominantly in the older age groups. The number of patients with a diagnosis of depression remained stable for males but increased by 15% for females, again largely in the older age groups. By contrast, the number of in-patients with 'other diagnoses' fell by 18% for males and by 12% for females. The decline was marked in the younger patients, with older age groups showing a slight increase. The diagnostic distribution was broadly similar in both years, with only a quarter as many patients in each of the diagnostic categories organic psychoses and depressions as those with 'other diagnoses'.

Southampton

The age distribution in both years for resident in-patients was similar. The proportion of females with a diagnosis of organic psychosis declined for the 75–84 age group. In 1976 the number of females with a diagnosis of depression was

TABLE 47
Diagnostic category [1] by age group – numbers of resident in-patients, 1976 and 1981

	Organic psychoses		Depression		Other diagnoses		Total	
	1976	1981	1976	1981	1976	1981	1976	1981
Nottingham								
15–64	21	17	68	61	137	127	226	205
65–74	29	27	43	39	30	44	103	110
75–84	61	75	23	22	25	36	109	133
85 and over	34	20	11	4	9	6	54	30
15 and over							492	478
Salford								
15–64	21	18	40	40	220	170	281	228
65–74	38	43	27	27	97	72	162	142
75–84	40	75	21	29	36	49	97	153
85 and over	13	28	3	4	8	14	24	46
15 and over							564	569
Southampton								
15–64	13	16	42	38	125	98	180	152
65–74	12	19	17	19	28	21	57	59
75–84	53	34	12	15	10	80	59	59
85 and over	24	17	1	3	2	6	27	26
15 and over							344	296
Worcester								
15–64	14	22	18	37	132	104	164	163
65–74	34	40	21	22	92	55	147	117
75–84	37	42	14	11	56	37	107	90
85 and over	24	13	2		13	7	39	20
15 and over							457	390

1. See footnote to Table 5, p. 16.

half the number in the other two diagnostic categories. However, by 1981 there was an even spread between the three diagnostic groups for females. The diagnostic distribution for males was the same in both years, with equal numbers of patients with a diagnosis of organic psychosis or depression; however, there were three or four times as many males with other diagnoses. Overall there was a 14% drop in the number of resident in-patients between 1976 and 1981. The number of males was approximately the same in both years, while the number of females with organic psychoses declined by 20%, predominantly in the 75–84 age group. The number with depression increased by 25%, mostly in the older age groups. The number with 'other diagnoses' fell by 35%, this drop being largely in the younger group.

Worcester

The age distribution was very similar in both years. The diagnostic distribution was also similar, although there was a slight increase in younger females having organic psychosis. The number of resident in-patients aged 15–64 showed no change between 1976 and 1981, while the numbers in the age groups 65–74 and 75–84 declined by almost 20%. The number of resident in-patients aged over 85 decreased by almost 50%. The total number of residents declined by 15% for all ages over the five-year period. The diagnostic distribution was similar for males and females. The diagnostic category organic psychoses accounted for a third of patients, and most of the rest were in the 'other diagnoses' category. The depression category accounted for very few patients.

Admissions in the two years before each census date

In general, the proportion of patients with a previous admission in the two years before each census date in Nottingham and Southampton was almost twice that in Worcester and Salford, as shown in Table 48. However, the over 85 age group was slightly different for Nottingham, being low in 1976.

Psychiatric care subsequent to the census dates

The proportion of patients in Nottingham and Southampton who were still in-patients after two years was half that in Worcester and Salford. The over 85 age group in Nottingham was nearer to that of Worcester and Salford in 1976 but not in 1981. In 1979 a Department of Health Care of the Elderly was set up in Nottingham comprising of both geriatricians and psychiatrists. This department took over responsibility for services for those over 65 for about a quarter of the register's catchment area, and, like the psychogeriatric service in Southampton, operates mainly by domiciliary contact. The proportion of patients with a readmission in the two years following the census dates was twice as much in Nottingham and Southampton as in Worcester and Salford. The difference was more marked in the over 65 age groups, but the numbers were small. This finding is expected in view of the proportions remaining as in-patients throughout the two-year period.

A similar pattern to that for readmissions was demonstrated in the number receiving day care subsequent to admission. In both years a much higher use of day care facilities for all ages was found in Nottingham, presumably a function

TABLE 48

Resident in-patients – percentages of each age group receiving psychiatric care in the two years before and after each censal date

	Previous admissions		Still in-patients two years after censal date		Readmission		Subsequent day care		Subsequent out-patient care	
	1976	1981	1976	1981	1976	1981	1976	1981	1976	1981
15–64										
Nottingham	74	66	35	31	27	32	24	24	41	44
Salford	36	40	67	60	12	14	6	7	14	20
Southampton	56	59	43	46	27	28	11	20	36	36
Worcester	32	47	62	50	13	16	7	14	18	25
65–74										
Nottingham	57	53	44	43	17	12	19	10	18	20
Salford	28	30	72	73	4	2	2	8	3	6
Southampton	35	51	40	46	16	17	2	8	18	29
Worcester	18	44	71	54	1	1	3	3	5	10
75–84										
Nottingham	66	58	36	35	9	2	12	6	7	5
Salford	35	39	64	52	1	3	–	1	1	5
Southampton	68	41	31	37	13	20	1	5	19	24
Worcester	24	29	61	52	4	3	3	1	4	1
85 and over										
Nottingham	28	53	43	20	–	–	4	–	4	3
Salford	21	22	58	48	4	–	–	–	4	–
Southampton	74	62	26	15	11	15	–	4	4	23
Worcester	21	25	51	40	–	–	–	–	–	–

of the availability of such facilities rather than individual clinical management decisions not to use day hospitals in other areas. Even when there is a deliberate policy of building up day hospital provision, several years may elapse before significant improvements can be made. Southampton showed a relatively high use of subsequent out-patient care, particularly for the over 75 age groups. The difference between 1976 and 1981 for those over 85 was very marked in Southampton. This probably demonstrates the effects of the increasing emphasis on domiciliary care for the very elderly during the period between the census dates.

The high use of out-patient care, with the similar proportion of patients remaining in hospital for a minimum of two years, and the higher level of previous admissions in Nottingham and Southampton compared with Worcester and Salford, may be explained in a number of ways. The differences could be attributed to population characteristics, but this is unlikely since Salford has an aging, declining population while Worcester has a younger, growing population. The patterns of care described may reflect the operation of a policy of shorter length of stay combined with higher levels of readmission in Nottingham and Southampton than applies in the other two areas. Further consideration can be found in Chapter 4.

Discussion

This study amply confirmed the expectation that use of psychiatric services is correlated with age, with people generally making higher use of services as they become older. The main increase in use was found among those aged 75 and over – the section of the community with the most rapid increase in numbers. Important trends, particularly in the development of domiciliary services, were found, suggesting that local psychiatrists are aware of the increasing needs of the elderly and are responding to them. Data up to the end of 1983 were used for this study. Since then the domiciliary services have continued to expand and the trends described have probably been maintained. However, closure of two of the registers involved prevented a further examination of the situation in 1986.

This study was concerned with the use of care provided by psychiatrists, but a large part of care is provided for psychiatric patients by other professionals, including nurses, social workers, psychologists and occupational therapists. Registers vary in their coverage of such work. Chapter 6 provides a description of the involvement of community psychiatric nurses.

The data obtained from these case registers can be used to describe in detail the patterns of psychiatric care received by patients; it cannot be used to demonstrate which patterns of care are the most effective or efficient. To do so would require detailed evaluation of the clinical and social outcomes of the various service options. For instance, use of day care facilities is highest in Nottingham, but case register data are not sufficient to indicate whether an increase in such facilities in other areas or a decrease in Nottingham would be an appropriate reallocation of resources.

What this exercise does demonstrate is that data from case registers can be used to illustrate quite strikingly different patterns of service development, even within the comparatively uniform general framework of the NHS. It also shows clearly that there are increasing demands over time; particularly from the very old. It seems wise to abandon the conventional statistical definition of the elderly as all those aged more than 65 years, and to insist on more detailed tabulations that will highlight the important differences in the service needs of the old and the very old.

8 A five-year follow-up of deliberate self-poisoning in Oxford and Worcester

J. DE ALARCON, J. FOOKS, C. HASSALL and S. ROSE

Deliberate self-harm by drug overdose is a major health problem associated with social deprivation (Bancroft *et al*, 1975; Morgan *et al*, 1975; Holding *et al*, 1977), family disharmony (Bancroft *et al*, 1977; Birtchnell, 1981), and other life stress factors (Morgan, 1982). It is most common in teenagers and young adults, particularly females (Hawton & Goldacre, 1982) and has a high risk of repetition and death (Morgan *et al*, 1976). So far attempts to demonstrate the value of psychiatric intervention in preventing repetition have not been successful (Ettlinger, 1975; Morgan *et al*, 1976; Kreitman, 1977; Gibbons *et al*, 1978; Hawton *et al*, 1981). Nevertheless attempts to prevent repetition by psychiatric intervention continue.

Controlled prospective studies to follow up patients randomly assigned to treatment or no treatment have not been possible, but the possibility of linking data from psychiatric registers to general hospital overdose admission records and to death records allows the outcome of those overdose patients who have had psychiatric treatment to be compared with those who have not.

The existence of a specialised psychiatric service based in general hospitals for these patients in the Oxfordshire health district and the absence of such a service (in the period under consideration) in the Worcester and Kidderminster health districts seemed to provide an experiment of opportunity, since both areas were covered by case registers, which could be used to measure the amount of treatment received and long-term outcome. We therefore aimed to evaluate the effectiveness of psychiatric intervention by comparing outcome in terms of repeat attempts and mortality in Worcestershire and Oxfordshire during the period 1978–83.

Material and methods

(a) Using hospital activity analysis (HAA) records we selected every person living in the two health districts who was admitted to a local general hospital in 1978 with a diagnosis of self-poisoning and who survived that attempt.

(b) The first self-poisoning admission in 1978 was regarded as the index admission.

(c) Data on previous and subsequent history for the cohort were obtained by different means in the two areas. In Oxford, since the HAA records are linked to psychiatric and death records by person, the data were immediately available. In Worcester, persons in the cohort were searched for on the psychiatric register and their psychiatric history, subsequent care and/or death obtained from this.

(d) The cohort is described in terms of age at index admission, sex, previous history of mental illness and self-harm, and latest known psychiatric diagnosis.

(e) Treatment received between the date of index admission and 31 December 1983 was measured in days by counting each single contact as one day and each episode of care as the number of days covered between the beginning and end of the episode.

(f) Outcome was measured in terms of mortality, number of subsequent self-harm attempts during the follow-up period and whether or not the patient was still in treatment in December 1983.

Services available

In Oxford a psychiatric consultation service (PCS) was available at the central general hospital in the city, counsellors were on call to visit patients, and ward staff were encouraged to refer all overdose cases. This PCS offered psychiatric ward and domiciliary consultation, out-patient care, open access to continued counselling and referral to all the other psychiatric services in the Oxford health district. This special service was consulted for 94% of all Oxford district admissions for self-poisoning in 1978; 5% were already in psychiatric care at the time of the attempt and 89% were new referrals. The PCS was not, however, available to outlying areas of the Oxford district served by two smaller general hospitals, nor was it available in Worcester and Kidderminster. However, even in the absence of a PCS specially aimed at these patients, all the above services were available whenever a psychiatric consultation was requested by the general physician.

Description of 1978 cohorts

Age and sex

Table 49 shows, as expected, that females outnumbered males in the ratio 2:1 and approximately two-thirds of the cohorts were under 35. Although the cohorts

TABLE 49
The two self-poisoning cohorts

| | Males | | | | Females | | | | Both sexes | | | |
| | Oxford | | Worcester | | Oxford | | Worcester | | Oxford | | Worcester | |
	No.	(%)	No.	(%)	No.	(%)	No.	(%)	No.	(%)	No.	(%)
15–24	50	(28)	26	(23)	141	(36)	74	(34)	191	(33)	100	(30)
25–34	65	(36)	42	(37)	105	(27)	57	(26)	170	(30)	99	(30)
35–64	62	(34)	38	(34)	124	(31)	75	(34)	186	(32)	113	(34)
65 and over	3	(2)	7	(6)	23	(6)	14	(6)	26	(5)	21	(6)
Total	180	100	113	100	393	100	220	100	573	100	333	100

TABLE 50
The diagnostic composition of the cohorts

| | Oxford | | Worcester | |
	No.	%	No.	%
Depressions	95	17	36	11
Personality disorders	67	12	33	10
Stress and adjustment reactions[1]	28	5	30	9
Non-depressive neuroses	18	3	27	8
Alcohol or drug abuse	47	8	11	3
Schizophrenia or paranoid psychoses	26	4	12	4
Other or nil psychiatric disorder	292	51	184	55
Total	573	100	333	100

1. ICD-9 308, 309.2-309.9, 313 (World Health Organization, 1978).

were fairly evenly spread over the three age groups 15–24, 25–34 and 35–64, there were small differences between the sexes and the areas. Oxford had a slightly greater proportion of patients in the 15–24 age group in both sexes; this may well be due to the large student population. In both areas males were at slightly greater risk in the decade 25–34, whereas for females this was a less represented age group.

Diagnosis

In both districts fewer than half of the people who made a self-poisoning attempt in 1978 were given a psychiatric diagnosis at any time during the five-year follow-up, even when seen for a psychiatric consultation (Table 50). Among those who were considered to be suffering from a psychiatric disorder, the most common condition in both districts was depression in women and personality disorder in men. Alcohol and drug abuse was more common in Oxford in both sexes, and adjustment reactions and non-depressive neuroses in Worcester.

Previous history

While the majority of self-poisoning patients had had no known previous contact with the psychiatric services, 32% in Oxford and 26% in Worcester were known to have had previous care, with no marked difference between males and females (Table 51). Table 51 shows that 21% of the Oxford cohort had in fact been admitted to a psychiatric hospital bed – a significantly higher proportion than in Worcester and a suggestion, since we know that admission policies in the two districts are similar (Gibbons *et al*, 1984), that the Oxford cohort was clinically more disturbed.

Previous self-poisoning

An attempt was made to compare the proportions in each cohort who were making their first self-poisoning gesture. However, this information was not available in Worcester for people who did not appear on the psychiatric register.

Table 52 is of interest in that it shows the value of linking with general hospital records. In Worcester, using the case register only, it appears that only 5% had made previous attempts. In Oxford, where all general hospital admissions for

TABLE 51
Previous psychiatric care

	Males		Females		Both sexes	
	Oxford (%)	Worcester (%)	Oxford (%)	Worcester (%)	Oxford (%)	Worcester (%)
None	68	77	67	73	68	74
Extramural only	12	11.5	11	13	11	13
In-patient	20	11.5	22	13	21	13
Numbers	180	113	393	220	573	333

TABLE 52
Known previous attempts

	Numbers		Percentages	
	Oxford	Worcester	Oxford	Worcester
None	429	317	75	95
One	77	15	13	5
2 +	67	1	12	—
Total	573	333	100	100

self-poisoning have been recorded since 1963, 25% were known to have made previous attempts, and even this is known to have been an underestimate when compared with evidence based on case notes (36%) or on interview studies (45–50%) (Bancroft *et al*, 1977; Hawton, 1985, personal communication).

Psychiatric treatment after the attempt

The psychiatric care received by the two cohorts of patients was compared after one month and after five years. Of all the Oxford cases, 94% were seen by the PCS staff at their index admission but few were retained in treatment and, as Table 53 shows, the existence of the psychiatric consultation service did not result in an excess of overdose patients being taken into psychiatric care in Oxford. Similar proportions, 13% in Oxford and 15% in Worcester, started an episode of psychiatric treatment within a month of the index attempt. (For the purposes of defining psychiatric care in Table 53, counselling provided by the PCS at the time of the index admission has been ignored.)

A comparison of the number of days of psychiatric care received by the two cohorts during the five-year follow-up also showed the services to be rather similar in the amount of care provided, with the exception of consultations in the general hospital at the time of attempt (Table 54).

TABLE 53
Psychiatric care within one month of index (excluding the PCS in Oxford)

	Numbers		Percentages	
	Oxford	Worcester	Oxford	Worcester
Nil[1]	465	259	81	78
Already in an episode of care	35	23	6	7
New care	73	51	13	15
Total	573	333	100	100

1. Includes patients seen by the PCS in Oxford but not taken on for care after the self-poisoning admission

TABLE 54
Psychiatric care during five-year follow-up

Amount of care	Oxford		Worcester	
	No.	%	No.	%
Nil	33	6	125	38
1–6 days [1]	354	62	104	31
7–30 days	29	5	30	9
31–182 days	69	12	36	11
183–364 days	40	7	20	6
365–750 days	16	3	7	2
751 days and over	32	5	11	3
Total	573	100	333	100

1. Includes patients in Oxford seen by the PCS but not taken on for care after the self-poisoning admission.

Within each area, men and women received similar care, but the services differed. In Worcester 38% of patients received no psychiatric assessment following their 1978 overdose. This applied to only 6% in Oxford, and twice as many patients in Oxford (62%) as in Worcester (31%) received brief psychiatric care in the follow-up period. The bulk of this brief treatment in Oxford was composed of interviews and counselling carried out by the PCS at the time of the index overdose.

Although there had been no excess of patients taken into psychiatric treatment in Oxford (see Table 53) it seemed that rather more of those who did receive treatment continued to do so for a prolonged period; 8% in Oxford compared with 5% in Worcester received treatment lasting for more than a year.

Outcome

The outcome of the two 1978 cohorts was compared in terms of mortality, number of subsequent self-harm attempts during the follow-up period, and the proportion of patients still in treatment at the end of five years.

Mortality

The mortality statistics for the two areas were unfortunately not directly comparable. Whereas the Oxford register receives all death certificates for anyone normally resident in the Oxford region, Worcester automatically records deaths only of those on the psychiatric case register. It was possible to check Worcester district patients with death certificates, and three deaths were found, but this was not possible in the district of Kidderminster. Thus while the Oxford study ought to include all deaths of patients who had not moved away, Worcester is short of deaths of some non-register cases.

Table 55 shows the known deaths for each area, broken down by age and sex, within one year (Table 55a) and approximately five years (Table 55b) of their index admission.

There are broad similarities between the two areas; both show a higher mortality risk for males than for females and an increase in risk with age, as would be expected for any group of people. Similar proportions of the cohorts died within one year of their index admission. Examining the deaths before

TABLE 55

Mortality of self-poisoning patients in subsequent years in Oxford and Worcester

Age range	Oxford			Worcester			
	Number in study	Deaths in 1 year	%	%	Deaths in 1 year	Number in study	Number with unknown survival
(a) Deaths within 1 year of index admission							
Males							
15–24	50	1	2	0	0	26	5
25–34	65	0	0	0	0	42	17
35–64	62	4	6	8	3	38	6
15–64	177	5	3	3	3	106	28
65 and over	3	0	0	0	0	7	2
Total	180	5	3	3	3	113	30
Females							
15–24	141	1	1	0	0	74	32
25–34	105	0	0	0	0	57	25
35–64	124	2	2	3	2	75	10
15–64	370	3	1	1	2	206	67
65 and over	23	4	16	7	2	14	4
Total	393	7	2	1	3	220	71
Both sexes							
15–64	547	8	1.5	1.5	5	312	95
(b) Deaths before 31 December 1983							
Males							
15–24	50	3	6	0	0	26	5
25–34	65	2	3	2	1	42	17
35–64	62	8	12	12	4	38	6
15–64	177	13	7	5	5	106	28
65 and over	3	2	67	29	2	7	2
Total	180	15	8	6	7	113	30
Females							
15–24	141	2	1	0	0	74	32
25–34	105	1	1	2	1	57	25
35–64	124	10	8	6	4	75	10
15–64	370	13	4	2.5	5	206	67
65 and over	23	10	40	36	5	14	4
Total	393	23	6	5	10	220	71
Both sexes							
15–65	547	26	5	3	10	312	95

31 December 1983, on average five and a half years after index admission, Oxford patients appear to have a higher risk of dying. However, the absence of data on nearly a third of the Worcester patients makes it very probable that the true Worcester death rate is at least as high as the Oxford one. The population over 65 is small and has a high expected death rate from all causes; including it in the comparisons seems likely to bias the results, so our discussion is based only on those under 65.

Although the numbers of deaths are small, making conclusions of statistical significance difficult, it is of interest to compare the observed death rates among our cases with those among the population at large. In order to obtain first-order figures, average death rates over five and a half years 1979–83 were used for each area to calculate the expected number of deaths in this period. Table 56 shows the results.

At first glance, as in Table 55b, Oxford cases seem to have a much higher mortality risk than Worcester cases. In passing, we noticed that the general

TABLE 56

Observed and expected numbers of deaths from all causes from index admission to 31 December 1983

Age range by sex	Population	Overall mortality rate per 10 000[1]	Expected number of deaths	Observed number of deaths	Survival not known	Observed/ expected
Oxford						
Males						
15–44	149	48	0.7	8		11.4
45–64	28	523	1.5	5		3.3
Females						
15–44	311	30	0.9	6		6.7
45–64	59	307	1.8	7		3.9
Worcester						
Males						
15–44	92	59	0.5	3	26	6
45–64	14	680	1.0	2	2	2
Females						
15–44	162	36	0.6	1	62	1.7
45–64	44	376	1.7	4	5	2.4

1. Mortality estimated from average of mean annual rates for 1979–83, multiplied by 5.5 years, using mortality tables for Oxfordshire and West Berkshire health districts for Oxford figures, and tables from the Office of Population Censuses and Surveys for Kidderminster and Worcester health districts.

TABLE 57

Characteristics of those dying within 5 years of index admission, aged under 65 at time of index admission

	Oxford No.	Oxford %	Worcester %	Worcester No.	Oxford % all patients under 65	Oxford % those who died	Worcester % all patients under 65	Worcester % those who died
Depressions	6	23	30	3	15	23	9	30
Personality disorders	4	15	0	0	12	15	11	0
Stress and adjustment reactions	0	0	40	4	5	0	10	40
Non-depressive neuroses	2	8	10	1	3	8	8	10
Alcohol or drug abuse	5	19	0	0	8	19	3	0
Schizophrenia or paranoid states	2	8	0	0	4	8	3	0
Other or nil psychiatric	7	27	20	2	52	27	56	20
Total	26	100	100	10	100	100	100	100

mortality rate is some 20% higher for all groups in Worcester than in Oxford. However, as mentioned earlier, since there are people in each group whose survival is unknown, the Worcester figures are likely to be an underestimate of the true number of deaths in that area. In any case, the mortality from all causes in these patients is consistently higher than in the population at large.

Clearly, we identified a group of people at unusually high risk of early death. Since those with a psychiatric diagnosis (see Table 57) formed a large proportion (73–80% as opposed to 45–49% of the overdose group as a whole) of those who died within five and a half years, we may merely be seeing one aspect of the general truth that mortality is excessively high among psychiatric patients compared with the general population.

The small number of patients dying in each of the diagnostic groups means that it is not possible to be confident about associations between any particular diagnosis and death following overdose. A comparison of the distribution of diagnoses in the total cohort under 65 and those under 65 who died might however

TABLE 58
Services received after index admission by patients aged under 65

| | Oxford | | Worcester | |
	No.	%	No.	%
(a) By those dying within 5 years				
None	0	0	20	2
At index only	7	27	10	1
More care	19	73	70	710
Total	26	100	100	10
(b) By all patients at the time of index admission				
None	30	5.5	117	37.5
At index only	315	57.5	58	18.5
More care	202	37	137	44
Total	547	100	312	100

TABLE 59
Known subsequent self-harm attempts

| No. of attempts | In first follow-up year | | | | To 31 December 1983 | | | |
| | Oxford | | Worcester | | Oxford | | Worcester | |
	No.	%	No.	%	No.	%	No.	%
None	484	85	307	92	430	75	294	88
One parasuicide	61 ⎫		19 ⎫		78 ⎫		24 ⎫	
One probable suicide	4 ⎭	11	0 ⎭	6	8 ⎭	15	1 ⎭	7.5
Two or more parasuicides	24 ⎫		7 ⎫		55 ⎫		14 ⎫	
Two or more attempts including a probable suicide	0 ⎭	4	0 ⎭	2	2 ⎭	10	0 ⎭	4.5
Total	573	100	333	100	573	100	333	100

suggest associations and is given in Table 57. This confirms that 'other and nil psychiatric' groups are under-represented among those who died, while patients with depressions in both areas, with stress disorders and adjustment reactions in Worcester, and with alcohol and drug abuse in Oxford, are over-represented.

Table 58 compares the proportion of the group receiving extended psychiatric care who died, with that of the cohorts overall. Almost twice as many of those who died had received extended care, supporting the conclusion that they were indeed more psychiatrically disturbed and hence at greater risk of early death.

Subsequent self-harm attempts

Similar problems apply to assessing outcome in terms of subsequent attempts as in terms of mortality. In Worcester, subsequent attempts were recorded only for those people who were on the psychiatric register.

In Oxford, however, people were entered on the psychiatric register by virtue of having made an attempt and having been seen by the PCS. Some subsequent attempts were identified by later general hospital admissions linked to the index admission and some by later PCS intervention similarly linked. Therefore again the figures were not directly comparable.

The comparison given in Table 59 shows subsequent attempts, and in particular multiple attempts, to be more common in Oxford, but this is probably an artefact since subsequent attempts of people not referred for psychiatric treatment were not recorded in Worcester. The 'probable suicides' include all

TABLE 60
In psychiatric care after five years

	Numbers		Percentage	
	Oxford	Worcester	Oxford	Worcester
Died before 31 December 1983	37	17	6.5	5
In care during last 3 months of 1983	46	18	8	5
Not in care	490	298	85.5	90
Total	573	333	100	100

known suicides and self-harm diagnoses on the death certificate. It is of interest, given the full coverage of attempts in Oxford, that 75% of cases do not repeat the attempt within five years.

Psychiatric care after five years

The least satisfactory measure of outcome is whether or not these patients are still in psychiatric care at the end of the follow-up period, since this is affected by local treatment policies and is likely to apply to a small but chronically ill group. Table 60 shows that there was no significant difference between the two districts in the proportion of self-poisoning patients still in psychiatric care five years after the index attempt.

Discussion

One of the purposes of maintaining psychiatric registers is to compare the provision of services in different localities and evaluate the different styles of treatment they provide. However, such comparisons are of limited value unless some hard data by which treatment outcome can be measured are available. In the present study we sought to evaluate the effect of a self-poisoning intervention programme by comparing outcome with and without the programme in terms of the amount of subsequent psychiatric treatment provided, the number of further attempts, and mortality. The two latter measures were to provide the hard outcome data.

Originally, it appeared that HAA and General Register Office statistics could be used to provide these data for both localities. When we came to analyse the data, however, we found that they were not directly comparable, the cost and effort of accessing all the relevant GRO and HAA data proving prohibitive for the Worcester budget. This problem did not arise in Oxford, where these data are linked to the psychiatric register.

We concluded therefore that, in order to carry out successful outcome studies using psychiatric registers, more data than are normally collected by the register are needed, requiring methods of accessing mortality and general hospital data such as record linkage or special surveys.

Apart from the methodological issues raised by this study, one finding of particular interest was that the service offering open access to psychiatric help did not increase the amount of care that the rest of the psychiatric service needed to provide. Further, even allowing for the probable shortfall in Worcester mortality data, there was no clear evidence that the psychiatric intervention service in Oxford had reduced the likelihood of further self-harm attempts.

Acknowledgements

We are indebted to the Oxford and Worcester case registers for the psychiatric data and to the Oxford Record Linkage Study for the file of linked data, and to Dr Keith Hawton for his helpful comments.

References

BANCROFT, J. H. J., SKRIMSHIRE, A. M., REYNOLDS, F., *et al* (1975) Self-poisoning and self-injury in the Oxford area. *British Journal of Preventive and Social Medicine*, **29**, 170–177.
——, ——, CASSON, J., *et al* (1977) People who deliberately poison or injure themselves: their problems and their contacts with helping agencies. *Psychological Medicine*, **7**, 289–303.
BIRTCHNELL, J. (1981) Some familial and clinical characteristics of female suicidal psychiatric patients. *British Journal of Psychiatry*, **138**, 381–390.
ETTLINGER, R. (1975) Evaluation of suicide prevention after attempted suicide. *Acta Psychiatrica Scandinavica* (suppl 260).
GIBBONS, J. S., BUTLER, J., URWIN, P., *et al* (1970) Evaluation of a social work service for self-poisoning patients. *British Journal of Psychiatry*, **133**, 111–118.
——, JENNINGS, C. & WING, J. K. (1984) *Psychiatric Care in Eight Register Areas*. Southampton: University Department of Psychiatry. (Copies available by sending £2.50, cheque payable to University of Southampton, to University Department of Psychiatry, Royal South Hants Hospital, Southampton SO9 4PE.)
HAWTON, K., MARSACK, P. & FAGG, J. (1981) The attitudes of psychiatrists to deliberate self-poisoning: comparison with physicians and nurses. *British Journal of Medical Psychology*, **54**, 341.
—— & GOLDACRE, M. (1982) Hospital admissions for adverse effects of medicinal agents (mainly self-poisoning) among adolescents in the Oxford region. *British Journal of Psychiatry*, **141**, 166–170.
HOLDING, T. A., BUGLASS, D., DUFFY, J. C., *et al* (1977) Parasuicide in Edinburgh – a seven year review 1968–1974. *British Journal of Psychiatry*, **130**, 534–543.
KREITMAN, N. (ed.) (1977) *Parasuicide*. London: John Wiley.
MORGAN, H. G. (1982) Deliberate self harm. In *Recent Advances in Clinical Psychiatry*, No. 4 (ed. K. Granville-Grossman). London: Churchill Livingstone.
——, POCOCK, H. & POTTLE, S. (1975) The urban distribution of non-fatal deliberate self-harm. *British Journal of Psychiatry*, **126**, 319–328.
——, BARTON, J., POTTLE, S., *et al* (1976) Deliberate self harm: a follow up study of 279 patients. *British Journal of Psychiatry*, **128**, 361–368.

IV. Future developments

9 The development of other European case registers

G. H. M. M. TEN HORN

There are psychiatric case registers in at least 12 European countries other than the UK. Except for the register in Eire, much of their work has been published in languages other than English (e.g. in Danish, Italian, Dutch and German). The earliest registers still in existence are those based on national in-patient records, as in Norway and Denmark, where data have been collected as far back as 1916 and 1905 respectively. The numerous studies undertaken using these registers have been summarised by Saugstad and Dupont (ten Horn et al, 1986).

A collaborative project involving the Norwegian and Danish registers, and others, will study sex differences in the onset of schizophrenia over time and place (Häfner & an der Heiden, 1986). The data for this project, available from the Mannheim register, cover a much shorter period, 1973–81, when this psychiatric case register had to be stopped, owing to legal objections raised by the Data Protection Commissioner of Baden-Württemberg. The National Icelandic Register, in which information has been collected since 1907, suffered the same fate. Nevertheless, both register teams are still active, not only trying to continue their registers but also utilising the data collected earlier. Part of the Iceland register is still able to function, using data from centres for people with alcohol and drug disorders. The Swedish Nacka-Värmdö register, discontinued in 1976 after a four-year test period, has been restarted since 1 January 1985, involving all in- and out-patient psychiatric services, for patients aged 18 years and above, of an area outside Stockholm of 85 000 inhabitants. In the field of geographical analyses (the spatial distribution of treated mental disorders), this Swedish register team has made an important advance with the development of a computer-based map analyses system (ten Horn et al, 1986).

Since the early 1970s there has been a national in-patient register in Eire, as well as two local registers (St Loman's and Three Counties), from which the prevalence rates, for out- as well as in-patients in 1982, show how largely figures can differ within one country (ten Horn et al, 1986). The Three Counties register has been used as a basis for investigating the apparently very high admission rates for schizophrenia in Ireland. The result is that, with standard techniques of clinical assessment, the rates of first admission are not unduly high.

In the Netherlands, the Groningen register, covering a population of 43 000 inhabitants since 31 December 1973, has, since January 1986, been enlarged to the total province of Drenthe, with ten times the population. The positive experience with the former small register, together (since 1981) with one in Maastricht in the south of the country, has led nationally to a proposal to replace the Dutch National In-patient Register (in existence since 1967) in about seven years by a network of interlinked 'regional mental health information systems'. There are proposals for a register covering the city of Rotterdam. Like the tradition of the UK register teams, which meet once or twice yearly, the Dutch register teams meet and prepare joint publications. Recently general practitioners have registered their contacts with discharged patients to supplement the information on after-care so far collected in the Groningen register (ten Horn, 1984), and it is intended that the enlarged register will play an important role in the evaluation of the results of an experimental 'substitution project', where a substantial number of mental hospital beds will be replaced by day-care facilities, to which new and readmitted patients will be randomly assigned.

One of the important differences between the Dutch and most English registers is that the former collect data on out-patient contacts with psychologists, nurses and social workers from psychiatric services. To what extent this influences incidence as well as utilisation rates will be one of the questions to be answered in this collaborative study.

There are also registers in Geneva, Poznan (Poland), Rousse (Bulgaria), South Croatia (for alcoholic disorders and psychoses) and Belgrade (for psychoses). Further details about their date of origin, population, type of services covered and results can be found in ten Horn *et al* (1986).

Since the need for more evaluative research became apparent in Italy, where the Mental Health Law '181' of 1978 laid down that hospitalisation was to be regarded as exceptional and called for a comprehensive and integrated community mental health service (CMHS), seven registers were set up in Verona (1978), Novi (1979), Albenga, Ovada, Sestri (1980), Portogruaro (1981), and Legnano (1983), following the example of the Lomest register set up in 1975. With their data, in particular about involuntary admissions, it has been possible to record how the law has been implemented. Since most of the new services are orientated towards out-patients, the Italians emphasise the need for developing a standardised classification of patterns of care, and are collaborating with other European registers to achieve this. Most of the Italian registers cover smaller populations (50 000–90 000) than the English, having been set up to monitor services in this size of area. Some results have recently been published (Tansella, 1985; ten Horn *et al*, 1986).

The most recent case registers have been set up in Spain. Beginning in October 1983, a register covering the Basque Autonomous Community, with a population of 2.2 million inhabitants, was gradually introduced, in close co-operation with the Groningen team. The first data analyses, including some 70% of the available services, show considerable differences in service-utilisation rates in different parts of the community and the need for improvement of co-ordination of mental health services (ten Horn *et al*, 1986). Three national workshops in 1984–85, organised in collaboration with the European office of the WHO and the Groningen collaborating centre, resulted in a second register for Gran Canaria, since 31 December 1985, and similar initiatives in Asturias and Andalucia. A register was started in Valencia in 1986 (Gomez Beneyto *et al*, 1987). The need for population surveys and field studies in primary health care, in collaboration with the local register, has been expressed by most of these Spanish register teams. Following the UK and Dutch example to meet once or twice a year, a first Spanish inter-register meeting took place in the autumn of 1987.

The WHO study of mental health services in 21 European pilot study areas (Giel *et al*, 1986) stimulated interest in the disparity of mental health services across regions and countries. Researchers participating in this WHO study, from countries where registers do not exist, like France, Greece, Austria, Belgium, Finland and Romania, have expressed interest in such developments. Information on mental health services in Europe, at present relatively scanty (Freeman *et al*, 1985; Mangen, 1985) is likely to be substantially improved by these developments and by the close relationships now being formed between register teams all over Europe.

References

FREEMAN, H. L., FRYERS, T. & HENDERSON, J. H. (1985) *Mental Health Services in Europe: 10 years on, Public Health in Europe 25*. Copenhagen: WHO, Regional Office for Europe.

GIEL, R., HANNIBAL, J. U., HENDERSON, J H., *et al* (eds) (1986) *Mental Health Services in Pilot Study Areas*. Copenhagen: WHO, Regional Office for Europe.

GOMEZ BENEYTO, M., SALAZAR FRAILE, J. & PERES BONET, R. (1987) *Registro de Casos Psiquiatricos de Valencia*. Valencia: Centro Editorial Servicios y Publicaciones Universitarias, S.A.

HÄFNER, H. & AN DER HEIDEN, W. (1986) The contribution of European case registers to research on schizophrenia. *Schizophrenia Bulletin*, **12**, 26–51.

TEN HORN, G. H. M. M. (1984) Aftercare and readmission. *Social Psychiatry*, **19**, 111–116.

——, GIEL, R., GULBINAT, W., *et al* (eds) (1986) *Psychiatric Case Registers in Public Health, a Worldwide Inventory 1960–1985*. Amsterdam: Elsevier Science Publishers.

MANGEN, S. (ed.) (1985) *Mental Health Care in the European Community*. London: Croom Helm.

TANSELLA, M. (ed.) (1985) *L'Approccio Epidemiologico in Psichiatria*. Torino: Boringhieri.

10 Some national and regional statistical challenges

P. M. WILLIAMSON

The philosophy of the Körner review of health service information (Department of Health and Social Security (DHSS), 1982) was to concentrate on the core of information that was necessary for the work of district health authorities, and their needs have properly had the main place in the discussions that have gone on since about the new statistical system. But those working at the DHSS and the regional health authorities (RHAs) also need the right statistics if they are to be able to carry out their responsibilities, and it may be appropriate to include here an account of how some of the present challenges seem from the perspective of the DHSS. Most of the paragraphs below are not about problems peculiar to the DHSS; they are mostly matters that must be of concern, in one way or another, to people in every part of the National Health Service (NHS).

Statistics for resource allocation

The statistical basis for resource allocation has been clearly visible since the implementation of the Resources Allocation Working Party (RAWP) report (1976).

The RAWP recommendations (now under review) offer a precise answer to the problem of distribution of NHS funds between regions. But they do not help in the other allocation problem – of how spending should be divided between different aspects of health care. There is no difficulty in identifying needs in the health field; the problem has always been to determine priorities.

Health authorities, in particular, have for the last 40 years expressed their anxiety at the capacity of the DHSS for identifying needs, and at its much more limited capacity for suggesting where expenditure can be cut. Indeed, this discrepancy between demand and supply antedates the NHS. About the year 1920, one of the first Ministers of Health told in this connection the story of the newly married man who confided to a friend that his new wife was always asking him for money. "Great Heavens!" replied the friend, "What does she want it all for?" "I don't know," replied the husband, "I haven't given her any yet."

This chapter was written before the division of the Department of Health and Social Security into two departments.

Ten years ago many of those working in the psychiatric services would have been tempted to identify their health authority with the husband, and their psychiatric services with the wife. But there has since been some progress towards the rational allocation of resources. Perhaps the first stage was the creation of the Programme Budget, published as an appendix to the "Priorities" consultation document 1976. This brought together the claims of different aspects of health and social services, and suggested various rates of growth (and in one case reduction) of expenditure; thus the total of accepted demands could be seen to add up to 100% of expected resources, not 110% or 150%.

The Programme Budget has been updated annually, but its usefulness has been limited by the ability of national NHS financial statistics to provide useful information about the allocation of costs according to client group. This is well illustrated in the case of mental illness. Figures are of course available for the cost of each mental illness hospital, and therefore for the average cost of a patient-week at these hospitals. The cost of a psychiatric unit in a general hospital, however, is less obvious – its share in the heating, domestic staff, laboratory, etc., costs of the hospital is not easily identified; so that in practice, the average patient-week cost is simply assumed to equal that in a mental illness hospital. Until recently most RHAs have been unable to say what proportion of their expenditure went on mental illness services. Statistical information, both financial and general, has now improved, and should improve further as experience with Körner is digested.

This improved information is needed by RHAs in order to compile their regional ten-year plans. Most of these plans set out specific guidelines for different elements of a comprehensive district psychiatric service, usually based at least partly on DHSS guidelines. The plans make fairly detailed proposals for development of psychiatric and other services over the next ten years.

Do the resource implications implied by these plans properly reflect local needs? The answer can only be as good as the available statistics. In the past, much planning has been based on the famous figure of 0.5 beds per 1000 population, for the number of acute beds needed in the new-pattern psychiatric services. This figure, which first appeared in the Annual Report of the Department's Chief Medical Officer for 1968, seems to have broadly reflected experience in a single general hospital unit. It was generally criticised at first as far too low, and perhaps served a useful function in the early years in deterring RHAs from more generous ratios.

Soon, however, it was found to be overgenerous. By the mid-1970s, many RHAs had had the experience of building a unit on this ratio and finding that a considerable proportion of its beds were never required. Here is a clear example of resources being allocated on the basis of inadequate information. In some cases subsequent inquiries showed that the admission wards that were to be moved to the district general hospital used fewer beds than the new unit provided, even when they were in the mental illness hospital, where average lengths of stay are known to be longer. More use of available local statistics could have prevented these mistakes.

Such changes have made the DHSS conscious of the dangers of oversimple guidelines, and the DHSS policy paper now suggests that "Each District must plan individually, in consultation with professional people involved". Nevertheless, some RHAs have sought to use the same bed ratios in all their districts.

This could lead to both overprovision and underprovision. It is hoped that work now going on into the characteristics of a community that are likely to raise or lower bed needs will lead the way to the use by RHAs of differential statistics to match their plans more closely to the actual needs of each community (Hirsch, 1988).

Statistics for policy formation

Ministers do not simply hand out what they consider an appropriate share of NHS funds to each RHA; they also have detailed policies about the working of different facets of the NHS, and seek to ensure that RHAs pay heed to these policies in managing the services.

So ministers also need statistics to provide a sound basis to policy. Papers for ministers' consideration and decisions on a policy issue will normally contain a variety of statistics designed to provide both a background indicating the context of the particular problem for decision, and more closely focused figures bearing on each of the available options, indicating the numbers who may be affected, costs, and so on.

Statistics may affect policy at two levels. Firstly, by illuminating the present position they may show the need for a policy initiative: for example, given the general aim of securing a psychogeriatric service in every district, statistics showing only a very slow rise in psychogeriatrician posts may suggest the need for a policy initiative to secure a faster growth. But at an earlier stage, statistical and other information would be needed for the decision that an identifiable psychogeriatric service is desirable. At this prior stage, statistics from research studies and other forms of information may prove more helpful than national statistics.

Policies are all too apt to outlive the reasons, and the statistics, that originally justified them. For this reason it is desirable that the statistical background of a policy should be kept regularly under review.

Statistics for community care

This certainly represents a current challenge, but we should perhaps regard this as just one particular current aspect of the more general task of policy monitoring. Where health authorities are seeking to implement a policy, such as the policy of care in the community, they need to be able to measure how they are progressing. Equally ministers, and under them the Management Board, need for management purposes to monitor progress.

This poses a particular problem where services have been reorientated towards community care. Mental illness services are moving further away from the hospital-centred pattern of most specialist care, so that the statistical pattern appropriate to other specialisms is becoming increasingly inappropriate.

Four main elements to community psychiatry have been suggested: general practitioner psychiatric clinics, community mental health centres, community psychiatric nursing services, and crisis intervention. Of these four elements, community psychiatric nursing services have been provided with a statistical basis by the recommendations of Körner Working Group D, but there are difficulties with all the others. Some of the problems are set out in Chapter 11. Working out a satisfactory system of statistics for community psychiatry as a whole is a challenge in which both the NHS and DHSS must play a part. Because the case registers can be more flexible than national statistical systems, they may well have an important part to play here. Individual registers are already adjusting the statistics they collect to reflect changes in the pattern of local services.

The search for the right performance indicators is one aspect of the search for better statistics of community care. Because of the diversity of existing services which results from historical factors (in particular the unequal distribution of long-stay in-patient care) it is not easy to devise performance indicators for mental illness that provide a good indication of current performance by districts. The present indicators provide at least one interesting new measure of the comprehensiveness of district services, i.e. tables showing the proportion of admitted patients (under 65 and 65 and over, separately) from a district who were admitted within their own district. We need to search for an equally satisfactory indication of the extent to which a district's services are meeting the needs of those who do not require in-patient care.

Statistics for accounting to Parliament

Since Parliament provides DHSS ministers with about £1 billion a year (at the time of writing) for NHS psychiatric services, it is natural that Members of Parliament should seek from time to time information on a wide range of different issues about mental illness services. Ministers need to maintain as regular, sufficient statistics to demonstrate the general pattern of services being provided. In addition, ministers will seek additional information, where this is obtainable without too great a cost, either in response to a Parliamentary question, or in the context of an investigation by a Parliamentary committee, such as the investigation by the House of Commons Social Services Committee (1985) into community care with special reference to adult mentally ill and mentally handicapped people.

Such questions may range over a wide variety of statistics with a more or less close relationship to the quality of care being provided in the NHS. Parliament (and the public) clearly wishes to have available information that is relevant to the quality of care. Mr Robert Maxwell of the King's Fund has pointed out that 'quality of care' cannot be measured in a single dimension, comparable to the business analogy of return on investment. He suggested six dimensions of quality that needed to be recognised separately, each requiring different measures:

(a) access to services
(b) relevance to need (for the whole community)
(c) effectiveness (for individual patients)
(d) equity (fairness)
(e) social acceptability
(f) efficiency and economy.

Standard NHS statistics do not go far towards measuring these dimensions in relation to psychiatric services. (Equally, as the Griffiths report (1988) noted, "there is little measurement of health output".) But statistics on particular aspects obtained for a particular purpose, can often provide additional illumination with regard to the quality of care.

In the long run, such information can often provide added justification for ministers' policies, or may alternatively suggest a need for some aspect of policy to be reviewed. Where this is the case, Members of Parliament can be relied upon to see that ministers are brought face to face with the evidence.

This short discussion has done no more than set out, without answering, a few of the main current national statistical challenges. We will perhaps at least have convinced the reader that the tasks for DHSS statisticians are not easy.

References

DHSS STEERING GROUP ON HEALTH SERVICES INFORMATION (1982) *A Report on the Collection and Use of Information About Hospital Clinical Activity in the National Health Service*. London: HMSO.
HIRSCH, S. R. (chairman) (1988) *Psychiatric Beds and Resources: Factors Influencing Bed Use and Service Planning*. London: Gaskell.
HOUSE OF COMMONS SOCIAL SERVICES COMMITTEE (1985) *Second Report, Community Care with Special Reference to Adult Mentally Ill and Mentally Handicapped People, 1984–85* (HC13-I). London: HMSO.
RESOURCES ALLOCATION WORKING PARTY (1976) *Sharing Resources for Health in England*. London: HMSO.

11 Information for planning: case registers and Körner

J. E. COOPER

The staff of several of the present UK psychiatric case registers have been involved in discussion with National Health Service (NHS) managers of mental illness units and hospitals about the implications of the Körner recommendations (DHSS, 1982), for NHS service data. Case register staff have no direct responsibility for the collection of information used for regular NHS service returns, but they became involved because they were usually the only group in the locality with experience and expertise in the large-scale collection and analysis of information using computers. The Körner requirements became a familiar subject of discussion at recent meetings of the UK Psychiatric Case Register group, and this chapter is a summary of points made by both technical and psychiatric staff of several of the case registers. For most psychiatric units and hospitals the Körner requirements present a new set of problems, since the previous Mental Health Enquiry (MHE) required only that a comparatively simple set of manually produced data be sent off for central collection and analysis.

What does Körner replace?

The Körner requirements, which became obligatory in 1987, can be viewed as a substitute for the hospital activity analysis (HAA), the MHE, and forms SH3 and SBH2. Together these formed an information system that was collected manually locally, and computerised by regions and the Department of Health and Social Security (DHSS). For psychiatry, the MHE was the centrepiece as far as centralised information was concerned. As stated in the first Körner report (1982), the DHSS decided to terminate the MHE "primarily for reasons of economy" (p. 23, para. 4.3). When the Körner committee and working parties set about assembling the Körner data sets in 1980, the stated policy was to compensate for the loss of the MHE by the specific addition of items of special importance for the psychiatric units and services. The final result has been somewhat disappointing for psychiatry, and seems to be dominated by what is regarded as appropriate for the acute medical and surgical specialties. Some of the reasons for this may be the remarkably rapid changes that have taken place in the development of psychiatric services, even since the Körner recommendations first began to take shape. This is particularly so for some parts of the extramural psychiatric services, such as developments in primary care, the accelerating expansion of psychiatric community nursing services, and the increasingly close links with local social service departments. It seems possible that the Körner recommendations also adopted the convention commonly followed by DHSS, regional and district administrations, of not including the psychiatric services when discussing 'acute services'. As will be noted later, the main specific extra recommendation for psychiatric services is to do with long-stay patients, rather than the acute general psychiatric services.

For many years it has been evident that the data upon which the HAA and the MHE were based were not necessarily either complete or accurate. At the level of local hospitals and units, these deficiencies did not carry any particular penalties, since the details of local budgets did not necessarily depend upon them. However, the recently imposed management system and the increasing financial restraints placed upon the hospital services have made it apparent that the Körner data sets may be used as a basis for strict financial budgeting. It is therefore very important that data collection for Körner data sets be both complete and accurate; without this, the Körner proposals may be dangerous rather than helpful.

Common ground between the Körner requirements and the experience of case register teams

Districts which now find that they contain one of the UK psychiatric case registers may count themselves as fortunate, in that the staff of psychiatric case registers have had considerable experience in the problems of computerised data management. They are also unusual in that they are highly motivated to obtain complete and accurate sets of information, for which they are responsible from start to finish. To run a case register satisfactorily, it is necessary to know in detail how to collect data and who collects data, in order to be able to exercise control over the completeness and quality of data input. The same team is also responsible for coding and for the input of data to the computer. Perhaps most important of all, the register team has the final responsibility for producing an output that is both understandable and useful. It is this interest and responsibility for the complete sequence of data handling from collection to output that makes the staff of psychiatric case registers particularly useful to those contemplating the implications of the Körner system.

There are, of course, some basic differences between data requirements for current service monitoring and the research carried out by case registers. The principal difference is the time required for useful data output. The essential function of a case register is the collection of a longitudinally linked record of the contacts of an individual patient with various parts of the psychiatric services; cross-sectional data are obviously of interest, but secondary to longitudinal linkage. This means that psychiatric case registers tend to work over comparatively long periods of time, and study long-term trends and changes in service utilisation and in the careers of patients. The intention of the Körner system is to provide useful service data, presumably available within a few months of the time of collection. However, it is quite possible that this basic difference between psychiatric case registers and service management data systems will diminish as computer technology continues to advance. The development of quicker and cheaper computers, with ever-larger storage capacity and new types of storage, is already significantly shortening the delay in the production of some parts of case register information. Developments in the use of linked microcomputer systems, which can also summarise and feed in data to the central larger computer holding the whole of the psychiatric case register, raise even more interesting possibilities in terms of rapid turnover and data usage. The staff of several of the UK registers are already involved in experiments with the use of microcomputers, and are discussing with the local service administrators the most useful applications of new systems.

Information groups

Stimulated by the Körner requirements, a number of psychiatric units and districts have set up 'information groups' which examine existing and required information facilities and resources. In Nottingham, for instance, the case register staff initiated this at the level of the mental illness unit, since it was clear that there was some danger of duplication of effort and overlap of function (and therefore wasted resources) between the case register, the staff of medical records and other administrative staff. The Nottingham Mental Illness Information Group was informal and had no official status, but it met regularly and kept a record of its meetings. Its purpose was to act as a forum for the exchange of information, views and advice; any person or group in the mental illness unit with an interest in the collection and analysis of information about services and patients could be a member. Representatives of the management, the case register, the hospital and community nursing services, medical records department, finance, and district headquarters all attended regularly and found it a useful group. Not surprisingly, one of the main items on the agenda was the Körner requirements and how to meet them. In such a group, it became evident very rapidly that those who worked in the 'front line' of the services and were aware of how information was being collected were often dismayed to see the purposes for which administrative and finance officers used the information. Conversely, these central users were equally surprised when they were told about some of the problems of interpretation of information which seemed to them, at first sight, to be simple and reliable.

There are probably two main reasons why case register staff have been traditionally more preoccupied with the completeness and accuracy of the information that they handle, compared with the administrative staff of the hospital services. The first has already been mentioned, in that case register staff not only collect and analyse the information but are responsible for the final output. The second is to do with the requirements of longitudinal linkage. Information that has to be added to an already existing record of a patient must be free from inconsistencies and every case register has built into it a series of both manual and computerised checks, to ensure that what is being added to the record of a patient is compatible with what is already there. This was not the case with the information required for the HAA, the MHE and other DHSS forms, all of which were based upon cross-sectional information in which the identity of the patient was unimportant.

Some special requirements of psychiatry

This fundamental longitudinal aspect of case register information has also highlighted some of the deficiencies of the Körner data set for psychiatric services, particularly with respect to extramural activities of psychiatrists. When a patient is followed through a modern psychiatric service, it becomes clear that the extramural components of the work, which have been prominent in the psychiatric services for many years, are currently increasing in importance, even more rapidly than in the past. For instance, in many parts of the country, psychiatrists are increasingly visiting patients in their home without being requested to do a traditional urgent domiciliary visit by the general practitioner. This applies to consultants, senior registrars and registrars, in addition to community nurses and social workers. There is an increasing tendency to see patients on primary care premises, and during such a visit a consultant psychiatrist may well spend a significant amount of time talking to general practitioners, as well as seeing patients face to face. Community nurses now commonly hold 'injection clinics' in primary care premises, rather than in psychiatric hospitals or in out-patient clinics. If the budgeting of psychiatric teams and description of their workload is to be realistic, interesting problems arise in view of the different sources of finance for psychiatrists, social workers and clinical psychologists. Even some psychiatric community nurses are now funded from general practice budgets. It is not clear how this increasingly wide variety of extramural activity is going to be dealt with by the Körner system. There is very limited provision in the data set (in para. 10.25, where there is a recommendation for a "code for location of the clinic"), but this is not adequate as it stands. This will clearly become a major rather than a minor issue in the presentation of the psychiatric data.

Special care will have to be taken about how psychiatric services describe their day-care facilities. The differentiation between day centres and day hospitals has been established in psychiatry for many years, but recent discussions among the UK psychiatric case registers make it clear that there are at least two, if not more, different types of psychiatric day hospital. A number of day hospitals have a clear bias towards group psychotherapy and comparatively long spells of care; others are designed to cope with all varieties of patient during comparatively short stays, usually in very close relationship with geographically close in-patient units. The staff requirements and budgeting implications of these different styles of day care are obviously different and important.

Unfortunately, only a non-specific day-care category is recommended, with subdivision within mental illness into 'general' and 'psychogeriatric'. Further subdivision within these for general psychiatry is needed, and there is an urgent need for agreement about terms and definitions if confusion is to be avoided between regions.

The basic assumption made by the Körner recommendations, that the new data system would be computerised, also set additional problems for psychiatric units and hospitals. Most district general hospital services already have quite extensive computerised patient administration systems for the medical and surgical specialties, but many psychiatric hospitals and units, particularly those which are comparatively isolated geographically, are not yet computerised. In many of these, there is still no sign of the provision of computerised services.

How can registers help?

Case register staff can probably be of most use to local managers as members of joint discussion groups with experience of dealing with computerised information systems. No doubt their first comment will be that it is well worth ensuring expert programming advice, as close as possible to the source of the data. If those writing the software and designing the data output are not aware of the meaning of the data, together with its weaknesses and strengths, the output may be misleading rather than helpful.

Another problem that needs to be addressed with guidance from case register staff is the problem of the crossing of administrative, financial and professional boundaries, so common in the psychiatric services. A unit manager will need to know what proportions of the resources used by a particular clinical team come from outside the immediate budget of the psychiatric unit (e.g. from the independently funded district clinical psychology services), or from outside the NHS (such as local authority social services departments). An additional problem is that clinical teams, appearing at first sight to have similar workloads and responsibilities, may in reality have very different ways of working and relating to each other and to teams and groups outside the NHS. Case register staff know from experience that, sometimes, it is only by tracing all the professional contacts of individual patients in a sequence that differences and changes in service provision come to light. Innovations in service delivery, however praiseworthy they turn out to be in the end, are often initiated only by ignoring existing rules and procedures. Clinicians who are innovators are often not the most conscientious record keepers or the most careful communicators, and every case register has its own collection of curious anecdotes illustrating this type of problem.

It may be, however, that some studies would have a more general relevance, particularly if they were concerned with examining the accuracy, completeness and validity of local service information when compared with the case register version of the same events or procedures. Validation studies of the new NHS Körner data, even if only on a comparatively small scale locally, may well illustrate some important problems of quite general significance, and would not necessarily take very long to perform. Extra resources, on a fairly small and local scale, may be necessary to carry out such studies, but a great deal could possibly be gained. The need for such studies will depend a good deal upon the speed of development of local budgeting.

Two developments are recommended only for psychiatric services, namely, an annual census of all long-stay patients, and the collection (if possible) at the same time of information about the extent of abnormalities in the "social behaviour or function" of patients (para. 7.6). To follow these suggestions will need even more effort, but should produce information of obvious local use. Dependency surveys of various kinds are a well known and closely similar activity, but their regular and widespread use should provide both interesting information and a useful stimulus for the production of improved methods of assessment.

In conclusion, it is clear that the Körner recommendations were a good idea in principle. It remains to be seen to what extent they can be extended to meet the special requirements of the psychiatric services.

Reference

KÖRNER, E. (chairman) (1982) DHSS, Steering Group on Health Services Information. *A Report on the Collection and Use of Information About Hospital Clinical Activity in the National Health Service*. London: HMSO.

12 The future of psychiatric case registers

J. K. WING

The new technology

Psychiatric case registers can provide information at many different levels and in many different forms – about individuals, about groups with particular characteristics, about service units or agencies, about staff, and about forms of care. This is done by using a wide variety of statistical indices. These functions are limited only by the quantity and quality of data that can be collected, stored and processed. Advances in technology mean that the size of the data base, the speed of processing and the flexibility of interaction between user and computer could be made enormously more powerful and attractive. But register staff have learned from experience to be selective, and to concentrate attention on the functions that registers are particularly well suited to. The advantages offered by the new technology must be exploited only insofar as these functions are preserved and improved. What is now called the 'human interface' has always been the major problem for register staff, both when collecting data and when trying to get the results of data analyses used.

Fortunately, a number of developments suggest that parts of the register process can be made more 'user friendly', whether the user be a clinician, a planner or an epidemiologist. Whether these developments can be linked in an overall system, with continuity from clinical assessment, treatment and follow-up, through unit and agency management, to general administration and planning, must remain speculative, but that the technology is available is not in question. It is not too early, therefore, to begin experimenting, and case register teams, because of their good relations with clinicians and administrators, provide an obvious environment in which to start.

A useful review of the problems involved in creating usable medical information systems is provided by Hedlund *et al* (1985). The following comments are less comprehensive and systematic, but they are based on experience of standardising parts of the clinical examination, of a needs assessment system for people with chronic disability, and of a case register that has been extensively used for planning local services.

Clinical assessment

Registers tend not to collect much clinical information, because of the difficulty of exercising any control over quality. The most unreliable item on the register

121

is the diagnosis, and more complex data about clinical problems and their treatment are not even considered for entry. Nevertheless, there is plenty of evidence that substantial reliability can be obtained. Self-assessment appears to provide a more accurate guide to the number of alcohol problems than a psychiatric interview. Carr has developed computerised interviews for the assessment of depression, phobias and problems of the elderly (Carr *et al*, 1981, 1982; Carr & Ghosh, 1983).

Standardised versions of general clinical interviews, like the Schedule for Affective Disorders and Schizophrenia and the Diagnostic Interview Schedule, are now well known. More complex systems, such as the Present State Examination (ninth edition) (PSE9) and its successor, the Schedule for Clinical Assessment in Neuropsychiatry, which provide symptom definitions, means of taking past history into account, and an aetiology/pathology dimension, are in widespread use all over the world. Making such systems flexible in use, and friendly in computer interactions, is only a matter of time. Greist *et al* (1983) have already reported a version of the DIS that patients can complete interactively with a computer.

Clinical assessment involves much more than eliciting symptoms, taking a history, and constructing a diagnostic formulation. It is aimed at providing a basis for deciding, at intervals if necessary, which of a range of medical, psychological and social problems require intervention. The ''problem oriented medical record'' (Weed, 1969), in various guises, has been intended to systematise this approach but it has not yet successfully solved the problem of the 'human interface'. Hedlund *et al*'s (1985) review is not particularly encouraging in this respect, although one or two examples of successful local application are given. Part of the difficulty is that the constituent items of the problem list are insufficiently well defined; part is because hand-written medical records are often useful and therefore used, whereas the computer equivalents are artificial, clumsy and omit the personal phrase that brings the patient to life from the memory of the clinician.

Recent experience with a needs assessment system in Camberwell has been moderately encouraging, although created purely for purposes of research (Brewin *et al*, 1987, 1988; Brugha *et al*, 1988). It is based on a clinical interview and clinical work-up using the SCAN system, and some extra schedules at interview to measure motivation and attitudes. Added to this are standardised interviews with key members of the caring staff and with relatives. The clinical researchers collecting this information then meet to decide, in the same way that a multidisciplinary team would do, what problems are present. Ratings from the schedules are used as a first statement of potential need for care but conflicting information has to be resolved by discussion. For each problem, decisions are made as to whether any of a list of interventions has been tried and with what result, and hence whether there is a met or unmet need for further action of a specified kind. The process is not automated but each step in it, apart from the clinical decisions themselves (which we think are not easily susceptible to standardisation, in contrast to the information on which they are based), is clearly laid down and could be programmed.

Research systems of this kind are not suitable for adoption in busy clinical practice but they contain the elements of what is required and could be adapted for teams working interactively with a 'clinical micro'.

A promising approach is proposed by Rohde (1986), a consultant psychiatrist with a practical knowledge of what can be achieved by using computers, who has devised a system based on his own clinical practice. The essence of his contention is that any computer package of this kind has to reward all the staff who use it, whether nurses, psychologists, occupational therapists, psychiatrists, ward clerks or administrators. The most acceptable reward is to provide up-to-date summaries that are clinically meaningful, allow scope for entries in free prose, make routine documents available 'at the touch of a button' that otherwise take a great deal of time to prepare, give rapid access to life charts and other historical material, and devise a very simple procedure for data entry and retrieval that requires no technical knowledge and very little time.

This system is, in effect, an orderly substitute for the medical records ordinarily kept by clinical teams. It retains much of their usefulness and reduces the chaos that tends to accumulate, particularly when an individual has made multiple contacts with a number of agencies over a period of years. There is a degree of standardisation; for example, the items chosen to describe mental state are based on PSE9 so that there are anchor points in the glossary of definitions, and lists of problems are provided. However, there is provision for free text and written records can, of course, be used to supplement the standard printouts. A prototype of Rohde's system (CRISP, the acronym for Computer Recorded Information System for Psychiatry) is already running.

The Körner data set and performance indicators

In Chapter 11, John Cooper sets out some of the difficulties now being experienced with the medical information system recommended by the Körner committee and now implemented in the National Health Service. The idea is excellent in general and contributors to this volume are likely to be highly supportive of it. But the long experience accumulated by case register staff suggests that this particular package has serious problems, particularly evident when applied to the psychiatric services. These disadvantages are all obvious from what has been said earlier. They amount to limited scope, poor quality, and difficult linking and follow-up. In one phrase, the data collected will often be uninterpretable. Registers, by contrast, have the corresponding advantages. They can collect data appropriate to local circumstances, they can apply quality control and, quintessentially, they know how to deal with changes over time.

A district medicosocial information system

Putting together the various components of the medicosocial information system discussed above might produce a system looking something like the one in Fig. 11, which is based on ideas put forward in Camberwell but could, in principle, be adopted wherever there was a conventional register and motivated clinicians and administrators. Information of good quality would be provided by clinical teams, using team microcomputers to generate their records. The teams responsible for a district would, between them, form a network that provided screened data to the register, which would be used to generate

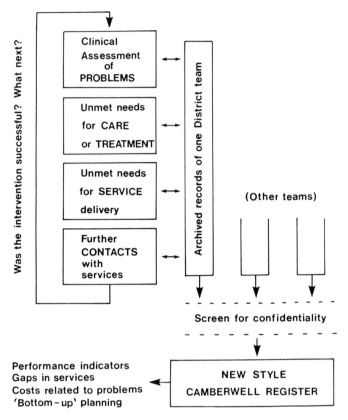

Fig. 11. A district medical information system based on the work of multidisciplinary teams using 'clinical micros'

meaningful indices of local administrative performance, based on the aggregate of problems experienced and needs unmet.

The problem of evaluating the accuracy of the assessments making up such a data base is no greater (and there is considerably more relevant research expertise) than that of making sense of purely administrative performance indicators.

The future of registers

Whether or not a system of this or a similar kind is established, there seems no doubt that registers, in future, are likely to operate in part by capitalising on information contained in computerised data bases, in the same way as most now rely on existing manual systems. One way forward is for districts fortunate enough to have a proper case register to invite its collaboration in implementing the Körner proposals. This would not only ensure better quality data but would provide a nucleus for developing a much better system in future. The UK has been at the forefront of development in this field and has the opportunity now to move further ahead.

The corollary is that registers, at the moment, are not being used to their full potential. Perhaps the peak of influence was illustrated by the book, based on the Camberwell register, to which clinicians, register staff and research workers contributed, and from which emerged the present pattern of services, now again changing (Wing & Hailey, 1972). Special local conditions, difficult to repeat elsewhere, made this possible. But the analysis, in Chapter 11, of the problems arising from the implementation of the Körner report, demonstrates that registers can play a substantial part in creating a proper basis for planning. This should be done experimentally. The principle of testing new and potentially fruitful ideas in a few key districts, before imposing them universally, is difficult to implement in practice, but it would save money, time and frustration.

One great advantage of registers is that they are not confined purely to hospital data but can utilise information from a wide range of local authority and other statutory services and from voluntary and private agencies, but this is not sufficiently understood or exploited by planners. The possibilities are illustrated by the comparison of the work of community psychiatric nurses and social workers, mentioned in Chapter 6. This is only a harbinger of the kind of work that might be undertaken. A register can only be exploited to the full if a team experienced in health services research is associated with it.

Several reports on psychiatric community care, including those from the Commons Social Services Committee (1985), the Audit Commission (1986) and Sir Roy Griffiths (1988), have emphasised the twin problems of the separation of responsibility for service planning and provisions between health and local authorities, and the lack of a proper information base on which to take rational action. They have not, however, pointed out that the two problems are really one. Griffiths (1988) asks for a designated minister with a powerful office and a substantial information base, who would control the disbursement of earmarked funds to a community care authority, which would be responsible for identifying and assessing needs, planning services to meet them, contracting out to agencies thought capable of running the services, and monitoring the extent to which needs were actually met. Neither the National Health Service nor local social services departments can provide the kind of information necessary to run such an eminently sensible system. Registers could, at least in designated test areas, if given the opportunity.

It is disappointing that, at the only level at which planning and administration for the health and social services could, at the moment, be integrated, the application of priorities resulted in the withdrawal of financial and moral support for registers precisely at the moment when, with encouragement and vision, they could have begun to take on a new significance for policy makers. It is not too late to remedy the situation if the main thrust of Griffiths' proposals is implemented without widening further the artificial administrative gap between health and social care.

In other European countries, as Chapter 9 shows, new registers are being established with enthusiasm. The underlying concepts are strong enough to ensure that some at least will survive to demonstrate the usefulness of the approach. Which country will be the first to appreciate their full potential remains to be seen.

References

BREWIN, C. R., WING, J. K., MANGEN, S. P., *et al* (1987) Principles and practice of measuring needs in the long-term mentally ill: the MRC needs for care assessment. *Psychological Medicine*, **17**, 971–981.
——, ——, ——, *et al* (1988) Needs for care among the long-term mentally ill: a report from the Camberwell High Contact Survey. *Psychological Medicine*, **18**, 457–468.
BRUGHA, T. S., WING, J. K., BREWIN, C. R., *et al* (1988) The problems of people in long-term psychiatric day-care: an introduction to the Camberwell High Contact Survey. *Psychological Medicine*, **18**, 443–456.
CARR, A. C., ANCILL, R. J., GHOSH, A., *et al* (1981) Direct assessment of depression by microcomputer: a feasibility study. *Acta Psychiatrica Scandinavica*, **64**, 415–422.
—— & GHOSH, A. (1983) Accuracy of behavioural assessment. *British Journal of Psychiatry*, **142**, 66–70.
——, WILSON, S. L., GHOSH, A., *et al* (1982) Automated testing of geriatric patients using a microcomputer-based system. *International Journal of Man–Machine Studies*, **17**, 297–300.
GREIST, J. H., KLEIN, M. H., ERDMAN, H. P., *et al* (1983) Computers and psychiatric diagnosis. *Psychiatric Annals*, **13**, 789–792.
GRIFFITHS, R. (1988) *Community Care: Agenda for Action*. London: HMSO.
HEDLUND, J. L., VIEWEG, B. W. & CHO, D. W. (1985) Mental health computing in the 1980s: I. General information systems and clinical documentation. II. Clinical applications. *Computers in Human Services* **1(1)**, 3–33; **1(2)**, 1–31.
HOUSE OF COMMONS SOCIAL SERVICES COMMITTEE (1985) *Second Report, Community Care with Special Reference to Adult Mentally Ill and Mentally Handicapped People, 1984–85* (HC13-I). London: HMSO.
ROHDE, P. (1986) *C.R.I.S.P. Computer Recorded Information System for Psychiatry. Draft for Consultation*. London: Riverside Health Authority.
WEED, L. L. (1969) *Medical Records, Medical Education and Patient Care: The Problem Oriented Record as a Basic Tool*. Cleveland: Case Western University Press.
WING, J. K. & HAILEY, A. H. (1972) *Evaluating a Community Psychiatric Service: The Camberwell Register 1964–1971*. London: Oxford University Press.